Indian Head Massage

A Practical Approach

Amarjeet S Bhamra

Nelson Thornes
a Wolters Kluwer business

Published in 2006 by:
Nelson Thornes Ltd
Delta Place
27 Bath Road
CHELTENHAM
GL53 7TH
United Kingdom

06 07 08 09 10 / 10 9 8 7 6 5 4 3 2 1

A catalogue record for this book is available from the British Library

ISBN 10: 0-7487-9608-8
ISBN 13: 978-0-7487-9608-3

Cover photograph: Massage by Corbis RF Zen (NT)
Illustrations by Beverly Curl and David Russell
Page make-up by Pantek Arts Ltd, Maidstone, Kent

Printed and bound by UniPrint Hungary Kft, Székesfchérvár

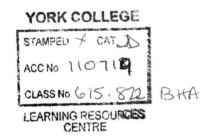
Disclaimer
The sole purpose of this material is to provide accurate information about the tradition of Shiro-Abhyanga, an Ayurveda-based massage application to the upper body. The information forms part of a dedicated course and many of the topics covered are elaborated on and should be expanded more fully during the sharing of this knowledge. The information is for educational purposes only and should not be used to treat, diagnose or mitigate a disease. If you are under the care of a doctor check with her/him the suitability for you of these suggestions. If you are seeking the medical advice of a trained Ayurvedic expert, please visit www.ayurvedabodywork.com.

Contents

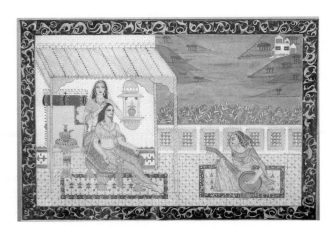

Endorsements

This book is endorsed by the following:

BCMA

Ayurvedic Bodywork
Consortium

The Ayurvedic
University of Europe and
The British Ayurvedic
Medical Council

College of Ayurveda

FICTA

About the book

Indian Head Massage has become an extremely popular treatment in the West. It is the only complementary medicinal art that is professionally practised by complementary therapists, hairdressers, aestiticians and beauty therapists. A state-of-the-art curriculum rooted in the ancient Ayurvedic bodywork tradition has to be universal in its approach and is vital to ensure consistency in any national standard.

What is Indian Head Massage? How and who does it help? *Indian Head Massage: A Practical Approach* is a commendable achievement in answering these questions. It is great to see that the West not only recognises but also is beginning to 'regulate' this ancient science of Ayurveda's bodywork modalities.

This book outlines how this increasingly popular therapy works, using case histories and diagrams, and provides a clear and comprehensive study of the therapy and all its possibilities for healing. Written by a dedicated expert, the work is authentic and gives comprehensive knowledge to practice Indian Head Massage with professionalism and integrity.

Dr Akhilesh Sharma
All India Ayurveda Congress

About the author

Amarjeet Bhamra is a dedicated therapist who has been working in this field for many years to promote this Indian treatment according to authentic traditions that go back many thousands of years. This excellent book of his is highly recommended to all students.

Gopi Warrier
Chairman
MAYUR The Ayurvedic University of Europe and The British Ayurvedic Medical Council

Acknowledgements

Dedicated to: my mother, Gian-kaur, late father Sant Kharak Singh
Bhamra and the universe through His Divine Holiness Satguru Jagjit
Singh the eternal guide.

A tribute to all my:

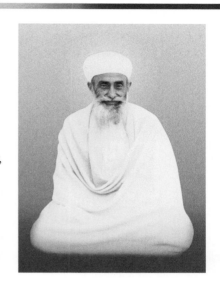

Patrons:
Maharaj Bir Singh, Thakur Dalip Singh, Thakur Udai Singh, Jagadguru
Shankaracharya Divya Anand Teerth, Swami Hari Prasad, Swami Ramdev,
Swami Athmachaithanya MD PhD, Sant Jaswant Singh, Swami
Indrananda, Sri Ram Baba, Sant Nahar Singh, Brahm Kumar Swamiji,
Bhai Mohinder Singh, Bibi Inderjit Kaur Khalsa, Swami Jashbhai Patel
Sahebji, Sant Amar Singh, Swami Gyan Vijay Saraswati, Baba Hardevji,
Pramukh Swami Maharaj, Anand Murti Gurumaa.

Teachers:
Dr Raghunandan Sharma, Dr Akhilash Sharma, Dr Suresh Agarwal, Leo
Angart, Sant Dyal Singh Namdhari, Tarpan Williams, Pandit Naresh
Saraswat, Acharya Navinderpal Singh, Alexander Barrie, Satish Shamra,
Howard Malpas, Dr Vasant Lad, Dr Jayshree Desai, Vasdev Singh
Bhamrah, Atreya Smith, Ayurved Ratan Dr Jagdish M Kaushal, Dr Robert
Svoboda, Swaran-singh Sian, Dr Deepak Chopra, Dr Keith Hearne, Ajit
Singh Satbhamra, Maharishi Ayurveda, Sri Sri Ayurveda, Anil Bhanot of
Hindu Council UK, as well as research on this book in magazines,
periodicals, books and the internet.

Associates:
Devi Elizabeth Wood IHM, Devi Claudia Ehler IHM, Devi Elizabeth
Brenan IHM, David Balen, Geraldine Scott IHM, Marie Rafic Abdu
Rjeily IHM, Marguerite O' Loughlin IHM, Claire Cullinane IHM, Mary
Treacy IHM, Joanne Coleman IHM, Noeleen Murphy IHM, Anna Steel-
Gibson IHM, Linda Graham IHM, John Murphy IHM, Cynthia Debono
IHM, Bassam Abou Faoor IHM.

Friends:
Devi Nina-kaur Sohal, Dr Vivian Nadya Lunny Medoco Cirujano, Caro
Ness, Palwinder-singh Bhamra, Ted Leydon, Brij-Mohan Gupta MSC
MA, Reiner Marcinkowski, Arjun Kashyap, Theresa Flanigan IHM,
Jayney Goddard, Bruce and Irene Hanagan IHM, Surjeet-kaur Panesar,
Julia Durrant, Pauline Rogers, Gopi Warrier, Anna Maria di Pasquale,
Varinder Sharma, Anna Maria Ganz, Harmohinder Singh Bhatia, Etienne
Regazzacci, Dr Mauroof Attique, Nicholas Rose, Jaswinder-singh
Bhamra, Sister Patricia Lynch, Joginder-Kaur and Paramjit-singh Neote,
Wrio Russel, Carol Lumsden-Cook, Susan Gleeson, Hely Abbondati,
Claire Jones.

HABIA/CSIA:
Members of Hairdressing And Beauty Industry Authority Expert Working Group for the development of the Beauty Therapy Standards for BT 20 National Vocational Qualification Level 3: Jane Farr, Tiffany Tarrant, Susannah Bingham, Marcia Henderson, Muriel Burnham-Airey, Louise Christie.

Nelson Thornes Ltd:
The entire publishing team with exceptional appreciation to Clare Wheelwright and Eve Thould for their un-opposed support.

Students:
With whom I have the privilege of sharing my humble knowledge.

And my special appreciation for the continual support and love of my wife Amrit and daughter, Aman.

A big thank you to Francesca Gould for writing the text features. Her contribution has been very much appreciated. Fran is Principal of the Holistic and Beauty Academy in Bristol. If you would like a prospectus, visit the website at the following address: www.holistic-training.co.uk.

Photo credits
The author and publishers are grateful to the following for permission to reproduce photographs:

Alamy/ Dinodia: 139; Alamy/ Jeff Morgan: 3; Alamy/ Mary Evans Picture Library: 12; ArkReligion.com/ Art Directors & Trip Photo Library/ Helene Rogers: 18 (top), 210 (both), 211, 222; The Bridgeman Art Library/ Vaidya Dhanvantari, Supreme Saint of Ayurveda Medicine, Indian School/ Private Collection, Dinodia: 9; Corbis/ Digital Art: 38; 5.5 Corbis GS V94 (NT); 5.8 Digital Stock 10 (NT); 2.01 Digital Vision 7 (NT); Dinodia Photo Library: 4; 5.12 Jules Frazier/ Photodisc 67 (NT); Getty Images/ Gary Cralle: 204; 5.7 Image 10037 (NT); 5.6 Tom LeGoff/ Digital Vision HV (NT); 5.13 Ryan McVay/Photodisc 73 (NT); Panos/ Jeremy Horner: 215; 5.11 Kevin Peterson/ Photodisc 33 (NT); Photofusion: 94; Reportdigital.co.uk/ Paul Box: 145; Rex Features/ Image Source: 18 (bottom); Rex Features/ John Powell: 144; Rex Features/ Voisin/ Phanie: 24; 5.9, 5.10 Nick Rowe/Photodisc 59 (NT); Science Photo Library/ Faye Norman: 11; Martin Sookias: 221; Superstock/Thinkstock: 44; Wellcome Trust Medical Photo Library/ Dianne Harris: 20

Shiro-Abhyanga

After working through this chapter you will be able to:

- have an understanding of the origins of Indian Head Massage
- gain knowledge of the history and development of Indian Head Massage in the West
- explain the benefits of Indian Head Massage.

History of Shiro-Abhyanga and development of Indian Head Massage in the West

Ayurveda is the world's oldest system of medicine and the forerunner to all the great healing systems. During the 18th century, Ayurveda was almost wiped out in India by the British raj who deemed it unfashionable and out of date. It was saved by Mahatma Gandhi who opened the first modern Ayurveda College in 1921. Indian Head Massage today is practised professionally even more in Britain than in India.

Shiro-Abhyanga, or Indian Head Massage as it is known in the West, is part of the Ayurvedic Bodywork series of treatments. In the spiritual evolution of a man, where Ayurveda is the body, Yoga is the mind and Tantra is the spirit. Together they form an interdependent trinity of life.

Massage is probably the oldest touch-healing art known to western society, but research has indicated that Westerners are reluctant to touch one another. Many people attempt to hide anxieties and fears within their bodies with the hope that the fears will remain a secret from themselves and the world. Eventually, however, they will return in the form of pain and discomfort.

> **REMEMBER**
> Indian Head Massage is also known as Shiro-Abhyanga.

Massage is a gift which many of us simply don't know how to accept. It is often easier to give than to receive. The ability to let go and allow a massage therapist to penetrate your essential being must be learned.

Massage in its many facets is here to stay and grow, from the most informal touching and cuddling of a hurt child to the highly sophisticated systems of Ayurveda Bodywork treatments. Over the years almost every culture has rediscovered the magic of touch for itself and formulated its own system of massaging and touching for health. When there are aches and pains it is a natural instinct to place your hand over the area, to touch a bruise or an aching muscle. Massage has developed from this instinct to relieve pain and discomfort. In today's society, the pressures of work, money and relationships have caused our daily lives to become increasingly stressed. In response, individuals have developed their own methods of coping. As a result, it has become increasingly important to find ways of dealing with these pressures that are both healthy and effective.

REMEMBER

Indian Head Massage may be given to someone fully-clothed and can be carried out almost anywhere.

Indian Head Massage is a non-invasive, fully clothed treatment that is ideal for clients who may be shy, such as pregnant women, the elderly, children and those with disabilities. The approach taken with Indian Head Massage is holistic. A detailed consultation is carried out, and a list of contraindications drawn up for the therapist to take into account. It is a 60-minute stand-alone treatment, which should not be blended with other therapies. After the hands-on treatment the client will be offered post-care treatment advice for improvements in their lifestyle.

During an Indian Head Massage treatment the client sits in a comfortable chair with the therapist working from behind. The therapist performs a flowing sequence of movements which begin at the shoulder and upper back areas, over the arms and hands, through the neck, ears and scalp, finishing at the face. These areas incorporate chakras, nadis, marma points, and vital nerve endings within the body, and so treating the head has beneficial effects on the entire body. The movements are based on a combination of effleurage, stroking, kneading, friction, percussion and marma (pressure) point techniques.

See chapters 9 and 10 for more information.

Shiro-Abhyanga

Shiro means mind, head and neck and Abhyanga means therapeutic massage. The head is one of the first areas that the foetus develops in the womb, and is the centre of the nervous system. The top of a baby's cranium has a soft area known as Bramand or the tenth gate. It sits directly above the pineal gland and the olfactory lobe in the mid-brain. The human body has ten gates from which prana (energy) can leave:

REMEMBER

Shiro means mind, head and neck, Abhyanga means therapeutic massage.

1 & 2.	Two eyes
3 & 4.	Two ears
5 & 6.	Two nostrils
7.	Mouth
8.	Genitals
9.	Anus
10.	Bramand, at the adipathi marma point

The Bramand takes about nine months to close. During this time, gentle scalp massage with oil may provide more prana with which the child can learn, think and memorise, and can benefit the five senses.

REMEMBER

Massaging the scalp will increase the supply of fresh oxygen and glucose to the head.

Indian Head Massage is a great treatment to receive at any time except for immediately after food and under conditions where massage is not advised. It is especially good in the morning before bathing or in the evening after having finished work for the day. Massage of the forehead and temples improves eyesight, creates a centred state of awareness, and increases concentration. Working on the scalp increases the supply of fresh oxygen and glucose to the head, along with the circulation of cerebro-spinal fluid. It also promotes the growth hormones and enzymes necessary for the growth and development of the brain. Shiro-Abhyanga practised daily can also aid scalp dryness, loss of hair and premature baldness and grey hair.

Indian Head Massage can be carried out almost anywhere, anytime, any place:

- Private homes
- Spas/retreats
- Clinics/hospitals
- Corporate offices
- Hairdressing salons
- Nursing and residential homes

Interestingly, in research commissioned by the Institute of Indian Head Massage, participants were asked where in their bodies their problems could be found. Whereas most Westerners pointed to their heads, those from Eastern cultures pointed to their heart region – the centre of emotion. This difference in perception, together with a western culture of complex modern technological lifestyles, creates a focus of energy in the head and shoulder region.

Thus, in this modern world, our heads tend to feel busier than the rest of our bodies. Our thoughts and emotions tend to constrict and twist the muscles of the face, head, neck and shoulders particularly. Sometimes we are more aware of one area than another: it may be pain or tension around our eyes, jaws, or chest, or back of the neck or shoulders.

This type of discomfort is the way our bodies communicate with us, letting us know that all may not be well or flowing freely. Releasing the discomfort not only eases the pain in these areas, but may also release memories, emotional traumas or visual images. Liberating neck tension allows prana to flow more freely between the mind and the rest of the body. This facilitates better connection between our thoughts, emotions, external habits and patterns.

The shoulders are often tight due to unexpressed or repressed feelings. When this tension is released, communication flows more naturally with more confidence and less anxiety. During an Indian Head Massage session, there may be cases when an old problem resurfaces. Ayurveda trains us to understand that holistic-based treatments are self-resolving, helping us to improve mental digestion dealing with our problems over a

> **REMEMBER**
> Tight shoulders may be due to unexpressed or repressed feelings.

course of treatment. Most holistic treatments that are being offered in the West are based on rediscovering Ayurveda.

Indian Head Massage: an integral part of family life

A healthy mind and spirit lends itself to a healthy body. As with all forms of CAM (Complementary and Alternative Medicine) treatments, Indian Head Massage is a tool used by therapists to help reduce stress and fatigue, increase mental clarity, and to relax and rejuvenate the client. It is used as a preventative approach to health and wellbeing. A lot of people are 'carrying the world on their shoulders' and this is where our stress, frustration and anger accumulates, manifesting as headaches, stiffness and shoulder and neck pain.

A variety of massage movements are used to relieve tension, stimulate circulation and restore joint movement. This helps to release emotional blockages and areas of negativity or stress, relieve tension, rebalance body energy and bring a calm centredness to the client. The treatment is based on ancient Ayurvedic traditions, which are found across all religions, helping it to be customary and acceptable without any conditions or barriers. This primordial curing art has survived through hundreds of thousands of generations and continues to flourish.

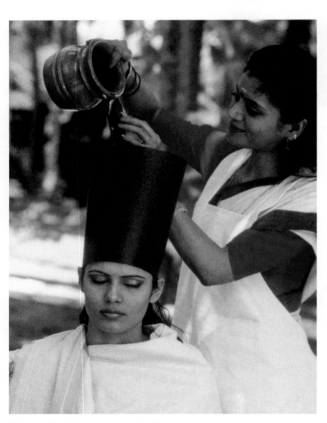

Fig. 1.02 *For centuries, Indian Head Massage has been an integral part of family life*

Almost every mother in the Indian sub-continent has practised Indian Head Massage, which has become both a customary and integral part of her family life. She may not hold a professional qualification or be trained at a college, but it has been a tradition passed from generation to generation. Using a variety of fragrant oils, sitting on her manji (hand-woven jute futon) outside in the warm air of the six seasons, she massages her family sitting in her lap at least once a week. It is customary in the sub-continent for every family to learn this ancient healing technique from their mother to pass on to their own children.

Indian Head Massage today

Shiro-Abhyanga was originally brought to the West in the 1970s by different spiritual guides from India. It has been in continuous practice since and like some of the better known CAM treatments, e.g. reflexology, aromatherapy, gained popularity in the mid-1990s. Indian Head Massage is now the most popular holistic treatment.

> **REMEMBER**
> It is traditional for Indian women to give regular Indian Head Massages to their families.

Unlike many other healing arts, it has made its home in a growing family of:

- Aestheticians/beauty therapists
- Hairdressers
- Freelance (on-site) therapists
- Complementary and alternative medicine therapists
- Parents who have changed their existing professions

No other treatment has had as much impact as Indian Head Massage in so many different industries and it is wonderful to witness the gift of touch being practised and promoted by so many individuals.

What is Indian Head Massage?

Shiro-Abhyanga is part of the timeless Ayurveda Bodywork system. Ayurveda is a holistic way of looking at health, i.e. a healthy body is necessary for continuous progress in life and can only be achieved if the mental, emotional and spiritual aspects of the individual are addressed equally. Indian Head Massage therapists do not treat specific ailments, but treat the person by stimulating and balancing their body, mind and spirit.

Indian Head Massage is a safe, simple yet effective therapy renowned for relieving the symptoms of stress. The beauty of the treatment is that you do not have to undress to be treated and no treatment table is required. A one-hour traditional treatment will usually include the upper back, shoulders, arms, hands, neck, scalp, ears and face. Chakras are also balanced at the end of the treatment.

REMEMBER
Indian Head Massage therapists do not treat specific ailments but treat the person by stimulating and balancing their body, mind and spirit.

What are the benefits of Indian Head Massage?

Particularly relevant today, Shiro-Abhyanga is a simple but very effective stress-busting therapy. It benefits clients suffering from aching shoulders, tight necks, tension headaches, eyestrain, anxiety, depression, sinusitis, insomnia, aches/pains, hair loss, sinus congestion, tinnitus and lack of concentration.

Who is Indian Head Massage for?

Massage for pregnant women, babies, children, couples, men and women, the elderly, the disabled and self-massage is essential to your total good health.

An Indian Head Massage exchanged at home after a long hard day enables partners to enjoy the evening together. It frees them from the tensions of working in an office or looking after a family that can often become overpowering.

Why do we hold tension in the head and neck?

When the body is under stress there is a tendency to jut the head and chin forward, which throws the body out of normal alignment. In an effort to balance the body, the neck muscles become stiff and tight and mobility is diminished. Shiro-Abhyanga relaxes the muscles allowing the neck and body to realign, which increases mobility and circulation. Toxins are removed and energy is able to flow freely between the head and lower part of the body.

How does Indian Head Massage calm the respiratory system?

Through relaxation, Indian Head Massage decreases the rate of respiration to a slow and even rhythm.

How does Indian Head Massage calm, revitalise and uplift the spirit?

By balancing the chakras and tapping into the Nadi and Marma Matrix, life force is able to flow freely throughout the body, thereby restoring the body, mind and spirit.

How is Indian Head Massage an antidote to stress and anxiety?

Stress and anxiety elicit the 'fight or flight' response from the body causing muscle contraction, rapid breathing, increased heart rate and redirection of blood flow. Indian Head Massage relieves tension in muscles, improves circulation, causes breathing to become slow and even, and can decrease blood pressure. In a state of relaxation, anxiety is diminished and the ability to cope with stress is enhanced.

Can Indian Head Massage cause injury?

Shiro-Abhyanga can be a light, moderate or deep-pressure massage, depending on the age and physical condition of the client, as well as the area being worked and the technique being used.

There are a host of exercises the therapist should be using to keep the hands and wrists flexible, supple and strong. This, along with posture and proper techniques, will alleviate the chance of injury.

How long is a typical session?

An Indian Head Massage session takes approximately one hour. There is a detailed consultation form to be completed as well as a list of contra-indications a therapist has to take into account and post-treatment advice after the massage. Indian Head Massage is a full treatment in its own right and should not be blended with another therapy or curtailed.

Unique features of Indian Head Massage

It is non-invasive, fully clothed, and ideal for shy clients. It can be carried out almost anywhere, any place, at any time and no special equipment or treatment table is needed.

Becoming a qualified Indian Head Massage therapist

Indian Head Massage is practised by a wide range of individuals, including hairdressers, aestheticians, beauty therapists and health-care professionals looking to enhance their portfolio of skills, as well as individuals new to CAM therapies.

Let down by religious, political and economical institutions, a renewed faith in the mind, body and spirit approach to health and wellbeing promoted a boom in CAM treatments, which continue to enjoy a healthy growth.

> **REMEMBER**
> Balancing the chakras will help energy to flow freely throughout the body.

> **REMEMBER**
> Indian Head Massage treatment takes about an hour.

Spas, natural health clinics and nutritional centres are being opened all over the world, and despite the often plush surroundings, the uniformed staff and enough certificates hanging up to look like wallpaper, these establishments may not be what they seem.

It is increasingly important that access to CAM therapies and the advice given to clients is both safe and appropriate. As the medical profession and CAM therapies move closer together, the ultimate benefit is to the client/patient. It would be a tragedy if the irresponsible, get-rich-quick merchants upset the delicately balanced prevention versus cure model.

Britain is witnessing an explosion of interest in complementary medicine both within Britain's National Health Service (NHS) and outside. Current development, particularly patient choice and local empowerment, will further fuel this explosion. Public opinion is moving the argument for integration of complementary medicine towards centre stage.

The NHS is moving away from the concept of citizens as consumers to one of citizens who are informed participants. One aspect of informed patient choice should be the ability to choose relevant options in addition to conventional patterns of care. As patient forums become active, it is likely that a wider choice will be offered locally.

Health and holistic living is no longer simply about keeping fit but has evolved to reflect lifestyle changes and now focuses on the balance between mind, body and spirit.

Progress Check

1. How long should an Indian Head Massage treatment take to carry out?
2. Which parts of the body are treated during an Indian Head Massage?
3. State four types of massage movement used during the treatment.
4. When was Shiro-Abhyanga brought to the West?
5. What are the benefits of Indian Head Massage?

Key Terms

You need to know what these words mean. Go back through the chapter or check in the glossary to find out.

- Shiro-Abhyanga
- CAM

Introduction to Ayurveda

After working through this chapter you will be able to:

◆ gain the underpinning knowledge of Ayurveda and its influence on other medicine systems

◆ to understand the five elements and the science of diagnosis.

Prevention versus cure

The Earth is a self-regulatory system with all the characteristics of a living being which has fanned the flame of ecological awareness and ignited a resurgence of interest in the 'earth mysteries'. The idea that a subtle energy or life-force permeates the landscape is an ancient one which is increasingly being validated by science. One example is the use of quartz crystals in computer technology to transmit electrical impulses, whilst crystals have been used for millennia as a tool for tuning into higher esoteric dimensions. Another example is the observation that the sea acts as a giant natural purifier of toxins, whilst it has long been known that salt is a cleanser of negative vibrations.

Earth is the element of form and substance, of solidity and stability, and it is by tapping into the vast knowledge of the Earth that we unearth our own deep-rooted instinct and contact the inner strength, the healing power, the majestic serenity, that is our human heritage. 'Do not seek to follow in the footsteps of the wise. See what they sought.' (Matsuo Basho).

Many practices considered natural, alternative or complementary hail from antiquity and are based on traditional folk medicine that existed in all cultures. Every culture and country had its traditional medical system, a blend of art and science with a generous feeling for magic, myth and superstition. As modern medicine evolved, science took precedence and medicine became mechanical, looking at life as a purely chemical or biological phenomenon. The human body came to be regarded as a machine made up of a complex collection of parts. Natural medical practices were pushed into the background and suppressed.

The human body is far more than a collection of working parts. It is a highly sophisticated organism imbued with the vital dimensions of body, mind and spirit. Most doctors are not always trained to recognise problems beyond the physical. Human beings are organic beings with a physiology designed to assimilate organic substances, not manufactured chemicals. Imbalance in mental and spiritual spheres cannot be separated from the physical, so how intricately are these interwoven? The healing traditions of India offer us a wealth of information in the practical matters of our health and wellbeing.

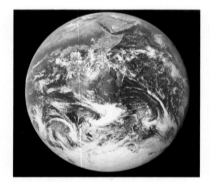

Fig. 2.01 *The Earth*

REMEMBER
Traditional folk medicine was a blend of art and science with a generous feeling for magic, myth and superstition.

REMEMBER
The human body is a highly sophisticated organism imbued with the vital dimensions of body, mind and spirit.

The oldest form of medicine, when considered globally, is Ayurveda. It tends to be forgotten that the materia medica of conventional medicine was, until as late as the 1930s, largely plant based and that botany was still part of the undergraduate curriculum in medical schools until the mid-twentieth century. Although today classed as a form of complementary and alternative medicine (CAM), globally and historically Ayurveda is the most conventional of all types of medicine.

Health is more than the absence of disease or injury. The World Health Organisation says health is a state of complete physical, social and mental wellbeing. Another way of looking at health is with a concept of wholeness. This means that total wellbeing exists only when our lives are in balance and we care for ourselves physically, socially, mentally, emotionally and spiritually. The spiritual dimension includes our values and philosophy of life, which gives purpose to life, an important part of wellbeing.

Ayurveda

Ayurveda is the natural healing system of nature. It is a manual for human health and wellbeing. It is a concept originated by the multifaceted Divine Trinity of Brahma the generator, Vishnu the organiser and Shiva the destroyer. Brahma promulgated His knowledge of the universe's natural health system through the chief celestial physician Dhanvantri.

Ayurveda (Ayu – age, life, longevity, r – relating to, veda – knowledge, wisdom, science) is known as the mother of all the medicinal systems. Indriyas: the five senses, Jiva, Atma: the individual soul, Manas: the mind, Sharira: the human body are the four components of Ayu. Ayurveda is prevention oriented, free from harmful side effects and capable of treating disease at its source. It is the most ancient complete system of health care in the world. It is described in one of the four volumes of the Vedas, the Atharva-Veda. The four Vedas – Rig-Veda, Sama-Veda, Yajur-Veda and Atharva-Veda – are India's most ancient books of wisdom, written in Sanskrit.

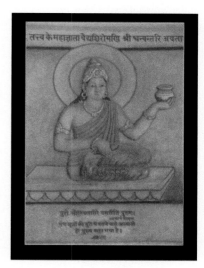

Fig. 2.02 *Lord Dhanvantri*

At the heart of Ayurveda lies the understanding that everything is one; that everything exists in relation to something else and not in isolation. It teaches that the mind affects the body and vice versa, that thought processes have physical effects, and that disorders of the body cause psychological problems too.

There are eight branches of immortal Ayurveda described in the Vedas:

1. General Medicine
2. Paediatrics
3. Toxicology
4. Spirituality
5. Aphrodisiacs
6. Geriatrics
7. ENT (ear, nose and throat)
8. Surgery.

Ayurveda embraces medical science, philosophy, psychology, spiritual skill, yoga, herbal and cruelty-free diet, dance, gandharv vidya (Indian classical music), Vastu Shastra (holistic concept of architecture and interior design), Tantra and Jyotish (astrology, astronomy and gems), and recommends a personally tailored lifestyle for a happy, healthy and purposeful life. It is a broad system of medical doctrines and practices, with both preventive and prescriptive aspects. It consists of a great deal of practical advice concerning almost every imaginable aspect of life, from cleaning teeth to diet, exercise and regimen.

In the West, the term 'diagnosis' generally refers to identification of a disease after it has manifested. However, in Ayurveda the concept of diagnosis implies a moment-to-moment monitoring of the interactions between order (health) and disorder (disease) in the body. For instance, in allopathy the concept of normality states that what is common in a majority of people constitutes the norm. Ayurveda holds that normality must be evaluated individually, because every human constitution manifests its own particular and spontaneous temperament and functioning. It promotes that a patient is a 'living book' and for understanding and physical, mental and spiritual wellbeing, it must be read daily. It teaches very precise methods for understanding the disease process before any overt signs of the disease have manifested.

Ayurvedic diagnosis includes some 32 pulse qualities which identify the condition of the viscera, as well as of the voice, face, iris, urine and sweat and detailed personal history including astrological aspects. Complex prescriptions are designed according to the kind of disease, the patient type, the anatomical site of the condition, the dosha dominance (type of element), the stage of the disease, the season, the age of the patient and a detailed consultation.

The influence of Ayurveda

For the centuries after the end of the Vedic era (5000 years ago), Ayurvedic medicine developed into a comprehensive healing system. Due to the various invasions of India, and the subsequent suppression of many original Indian ways of life, several ancient texts have been stolen and destroyed, but through the continued Guru/student relationship, enough have survived to ensure the active continuation of these highly valued, greatly respected teachings.

Ayurveda's theoretical foundation is a doctrine of three bodily humours (wind, bile and phlegm), somewhat analogous to the more recent Greek teaching of Hippocrates and Galen. In turn, Greek medicine strongly influenced the subsequent development of allopathic (western) medicine. However, the question remains by how much or to what degree Ayurveda has influenced current techniques.

The five elements in Chinese medicine were brought to China by Indian Buddhist missionaries, many of whom were skilled Ayurvedic practitioners. The missionaries originated the famous silk route from China through Persia to the Middle East influencing the people of these lands. Unani medicine, for example, is an intricate mix of Ayurvedic practices and philosophy with an Islamic shamanic influence.

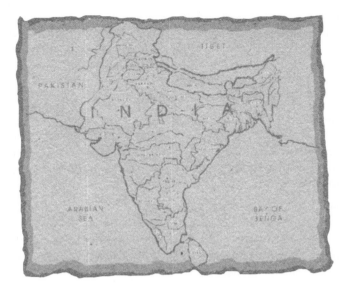

Fig. 2.03 *India, the birth place of Ayurveda*

Tri-doshas

Like other traditional systems, the essence of Ayurveda is balance between all the constituents, qualities and energies, within and without. In creating Ayurveda as a healing system, these elements were described in a simplified form as three vital energies or doshas. Each dosha is a combination of two elements. The three doshas are believed to be responsible for all the physiological and psychological processes in our body and mind. They are dynamic forces that determine growth and decay. Each of our physical characteristics, mental capacities and emotional tendencies can be described in terms of the three doshas.

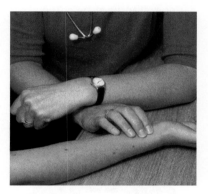

Fig. 2.04 *Taking a pulse reading*

Dosha means 'that which changes'. It is a word derived from the root dus, which is equivalent to the English prefix dys- such as in dysfunction, dystrophy, etc. In this sense, dosha can be regarded as a fault, mistake, error or a transgression against the cosmic rhythm. The doshas are constantly moving in dynamic balance, one with the others. Evaluation of the tri (three) dosha is conducted from the pulse in the client's radial artery.

There are five basic elements that represent five states or qualities of energy or matter:

1. Earth
    Earth does not equate to the literal meaning of earth, but to the force behind the solidity, cohesion and compactness. Earth is heavy and occupies space. It is reliable, stable, offers nurture and supports immune functions.

2. Water
    Water equates to the force that keeps matter in a liquid or flowing form, of fluids. Water is cohesive and cold. It cleans and dissolves negativity as well as preserving and protecting our memories. Kapa is earth and water combined as mucus.

3. Fire
Fire is simply the power to change or transmute the state of substance: digestion, metabolism and adaptation. Fire is hot and sharp. It allows the mind to control our emotions through perception and transforming.
Pita is fire and water combined as bile.

4. Air/Wind
Air/wind relates to power behind movement, sensation, the nervous system and animation. Air is cold and light. It governs movement and our emotional and mental impulses. It represents the vital breath.

5. Space
Space/ether is the field that is simultaneously the source of all matter and the space in which it exists. Ether is spacious and is the prevalent subtle energy in which the cosmos vibrates. Vata is air and space combined as gases.

Ayurveda provides a model to look at each individual as a unique make up of the three doshas and to thereby design treatment protocols that specifically address an individual's health challenges. When any of the doshas become dominant, Ayurveda will suggest specific lifestyle and nutritional guidelines to assist the individual in reducing the dosha that has become excessive. Ayurvedic practitioners believe that people become unwell when the balance among the doshas is disrupted.

Prakriti
Doshas regulate all physical and psychological behaviours, from basic cell structure to the most complex mental functions. The doshas are found in unique proportions in every individual. This unique combination of the doshas is called our prakriti, our natural constitution or spiritual DNA, and it will determine our basic physical appearance, preferences, behaviour and emotional tendencies. We are born with a body type which is unique to us and which we cannot change. Ancestors, parents and developmental factors in the womb determine this natal constitution. In Ayurveda, the diagnosis of disease and individual constitution is done by balancing the doshas. Prakriti represents the proportion of the three doshas and three gunas (attitudes). It is that very proportion which manifests in the physical and psychological features of that person.

Vikriti
Vikriti or doshic vitation refers to the degree to which an individual has deviated from the original proportion of the three doshas (prakriti).

Characteristics of body types

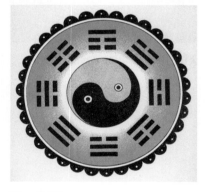

Fig. 2.05

Table 2.01 *Characteristics of body types*

Physical traits	Vata	Pita	Kapa
Resting pulse (bpm)	80–100	70–80	60–70
Body frame	☐ Thin	☐ Medium	☐ Large
Weight	☐ Low or bony	☐ Medium or muscular	☐ Gain easily
Frame	☐ Thin, poor physique	☐ Medium, moderate	☐ Stout, large
Hair	☐ Dry, wiry	☐ Soft, early grey, bald	☐ Oily, thick, lustrous
Eyebrows	☐ Small, fine	☐ Moderate, fine	☐ Bushy, thick
Eyes	☐ Small, brown	☐ Medium, blue/green	☐ Wide, black
Nose	☐ Small, thin, crooked	☐ Medium	☐ Large, firm, oily
Lips	☐ Small, thin, dry	☐ Medium, soft, red	☐ Thick, firm, smooth
Voice	☐ Low or weak	☐ High or sharp	☐ Slow or silent
Appetite	☐ Variable, erratic	☐ Strong/sharp	☐ Constant or low
Complexion	☐ Shady, dull	☐ Glowing	☐ Pale
Fingernails	☐ Cracking, thin	☐ Soft, pink, medium	☐ Wide, white, thick
Pulse	☐ Rapid	☐ Moderate	☐ Slow
Hands	☐ Small, cold	☐ Medium, warm, pink	☐ Large, thick, cool
Skin	☐ Dry, thin, rough	☐ Warm, soft, moles	☐ Moist, thick, smooth
Body odour	☐ Scanty, rare odour	☐ Strong odour	☐ Moderate
Bowel movement	☐ Scanty, constipated	☐ Abundant, diarrhoea	☐ Moderate, solid
Habits	☐ Artistic, dancing	☐ Politics, sport	☐ Selling, business
Action	☐ Unsteady, fast	☐ Goal seeking, purposeful	☐ Stately, steady, slow
Resistance to disease	☐ Weak immunity	☐ Prone to infections	☐ Good resistance
Which bothers you most?	☐ Cold and dry	☐ Sun and heat	☐ Cold and damp
Energy	☐ Comes in bursts	☐ Average stamina	☐ Good endurance
Body totals	**Vata**	**Pita**	**Kapa**
Mental traits	**Vata**	**Pita**	**Kapa**
Mental nature	☐ Quick, indecisive	☐ Perfectionist, critical	☐ Slow, stable
Memory	☐ Quick to learn, soon forgets	☐ Sharp or clear	☐ Slow to learn, never forgets
Moods	☐ Change quickly	☐ Change slowly	☐ Unchanging
Dreams	☐ Flying or anxious	☐ Fighting or in colour	☐ Few or romantic
Temperament	☐ Nervous or fearful	☐ Irritable or impatient	☐ Easy going
Speech	☐ Quick or talkative	☐ Moderate or argues	☐ Slow or silent
Habits	☐ Travel or nature	☐ Ambitious, perfectionist	☐ Calm, cool
Emotions	☐ Enthusiastic or worries	☐ Warm or angry	☐ Calm or attached
Beliefs	☐ Radical or changing	☐ Leader or goal oriented	☐ Loyal or constant
Mind totals	**Vata**	**Pita**	**Kapa**

The highest of the three totals indicates the fundamental principle that you most need to balance. The Vata, Pita and Kapa self-analysis will help you to identify simple changes in your diet or daily routine which may help you to stay fit and healthy. For example, if Vata is your highest score then choose Vata foods and consider other measures to help keep Vata in balance. If two columns have almost the same totals, then you should try to balance both doshas.

Progress Check

1. What does Ayurveda mean?
2. What is CAM?
3. What is the World Health Organisation's definition of health?
4. What are Vedas?
5. What are the five basic elements that are condensed to represent tri-doshas?

> **REMEMBER**
>
> **Vata**
> Space/Air
> Gases
>
> **Pita**
> Fire/Water
> Bile
>
> **Kapa**
> Water/Earth
> Mucus

Vata (Space/Air)

Vata is known as the moving force. It is mainly concerned with the nervous system and bodily movement. It chews and swallows food, moves nutrients and waste into and out of cells, circulates blood and air, and retrieves and stores memories.

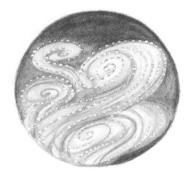

Fig. 2.06 *Vata*

Vata imbalance of modern life

Junk food, stale food, chemicals, drugs, video screens, travel, desk jobs, air-conditioning and most modern technology all increase Vata. This is because of excessive mental activity and reduction of physical activity. Many people will have an apparent Vata imbalance detectable in their pulse. Vata is aggravated by mental stress, fast-paced life, too much travel, positive ions in the air, synthetic radiation, technology, drugs and stale supermarket food. The symptoms of Vata imbalance include insomnia, stiffness, restricted movement, clogged channel (constipation), channels flowing too fast (diarrhoea), mental illness, fear, lower bowel problems, being forgetful, irrational and inconsistent behaviour, rapid highs and lows, grey and dried appearance.

> **REMEMBER**
>
> Junk food, stale food, chemicals, drugs, video screens, travel, desk jobs, air conditioning and most modern technology all increase Vata.

When in balance:

Vibrant, lively, enthusiastic, clear, alert mind, flexible, exhilarated, imaginative, sensitive, talkative and quick to respond.

When out of balance:

Restless, unsettled, light interrupted sleep, tendency to over exert, fatigued, constipated, anxious, worried and underweight.

What aggravates Vata?

Irregular routine, staying up late, irregular meals, cold, dry weather, excessive mental work, travelling, injury and too much bitter, astringent or pungent food.

Remedies for Vata

Exercise – gentle, moderate, regular yoga
Tastes – sweet, sour, salty
Foods – warm, mildly spiced foods eaten at set times. Refrain from cold/raw foods and cold desserts.

Pita (Fire/Water)

Fig. 2.07 *Pita*

Pita governs biological fire and is mainly concerned with the body's balance of kinetic and potential energies. Pita's processes involve digestion, whether it is digestion of food and nutrients or digestion of thoughts and theories in the mind.

When in balance:

Warm, loving, contented, enjoys challenges, strong digestion, lustrous complexion, good concentration, articulate and precise speech, courageous, sharp wit and intellectual.

When out of balance:

Demanding, perfectionist, predisposition towards frustration, anger, tendency towards skin rashes, irritable, impatient, prematurely grey hair and early hair loss.

What aggravates Pita?

Excessive heat or exposure to the sun, alcohol, smoking, time pressure, deadlines, pharmaceutical drugs (especially antibiotics), indigestion, excessive activity, and too much spicy, sour or salty food, skipping meals.

Remedies for Pita

    Exercise – moderate, non-competitive yoga and water or winter sports
    Tastes – sweet, bitter, astringent
    Foods – cool to warm mildly spiced foods. Refrain from salty, hot, spicy and oily foods, sour fruit, yoghurt, tomatoes and vinegar.

Kapa (Water/Earth)

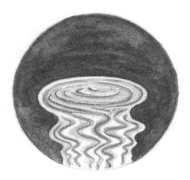

Fig. 2.08 *Kapa*

Kapa gives us substance/support and is mainly concerned with providing the physical field for the Vata and Pita energies. It governs cell structure, bodily secretions, and gives the mind stability.

When in balance:

Affectionate, compassionate, forgiving, emotionally steady, relaxed, slow, methodical, good memory, good stamina, stability, and natural resistance to sickness.

When out of balance:

Complacent, dull, oily skin, allergies, slow digestion, lethargic, possessive, over-attached, tendency to oversleep and overweight.

What aggravates Kapa:

Excessive rest and oversleeping, doubts, greed, lack of compassion, doing nothing, over-eating, insufficient exercise, too little variety in life, heavy, oily foods, fats, dairy produce, too much sweet (chocolate), sour or salty foods and cold, wet weather.

Remedies for Kapa

    Exercise – regular, vigorous yoga
    Tastes – pungent, bitter, astringent
    Foods – warm, light foods. Refrain from heavy and iced foods, dairy and iced drinks and sweets.

When altering the doshas one can learn to adjust so as to reduce distortions, prevent imbalances and treat them when necessary. Knowing your own constitution thus allows you to understand the workings of your mind and body better, thereby allowing greater control over the traits through planned and adequate changes incorporated into your lifestyle. A little time each day spent on your health may prevent a long time one day spent with illness.

Srotas (web-like connections of physiological factors)

As explained in Ayurveda 'people do not get sick from disease, but rather diseases reflect a disruption in the dynamic balance between themselves and their environment'. Ayurveda views the human body as being composed of innumerable channels that supply nutrients to the various tissues of the body. These channels are known as Srotas in Sanskrit, from the word 'sru' meaning 'to flow'. The body is likened to a system of canals which serve to nourish the different tissues and organs. Three key notions help us illustrate and organise the web-like thinking that is essential to the success of the Ayurvedic medical practitioners.

1. The antecedents of our patients' dysfunction nest within their biological terrain and genetic susceptibilities.
2. The patient's dynamic balance has constant perturbations that require adaptation.
3. Some trigger forces such as allergens, xenobiotics, drugs, endotoxins and emotional stress are strong enough to create a dysfunctional response.

There are many research studies that demonstrate a link or susceptibility to dysfunction between the environment, diet and lifestyle and the individual. The interaction of the internal environment of the individual and the external environment of nature is brought about by these web-like connections, described by the ancient sages as Srotas.

Tri-Gunas

The three influential principles, which regulate and govern environmental and biological processes, emanate from primordial nature pervading the universe in every human being, though varying in proportion. The Sanskrit word for this is guna – an influence that regulates cosmic forces.

1. Satvic (sat = truth, purity, knowledge, joy, being) contributes to mental illumination, general wellbeing, easy ability to adapt to circumstances, clarity of purpose, appreciation of order, refinement of the body and personality, and progressive spiritual growth.
2. Rajasic (raj = active, desire, restlessness, dynamically active) contributes to goal-oriented endeavour, resistance to contrary conditions, attempts to dominate, assertion of will, inclination to create and aspire.
3. Tamasic (tam = inaction, delusion, dullness to decline or perish) contributes to clouded mental faculties, confusion, delusion, emotional heaviness, laziness, indifference to change and new experiences, and unconsciousness. It opposes the influences of both Satvic and Rajasic gunas.

These three gunas are the basic constituents of prakriti (nature). With rigorous practice, devotion and determination, we can become our satvic nature. Through the sincere, dedicated practice of a Vedic lifestyle, a person can transcend these gunas and become free from samsara.

Dhatus

The Sapta (seven) Dhatus (tissues) elements form the pillars of the body that form the means of nourishment and growth while providing support to the body as well as the mind.

1. Rasa (fluid) Dhatu – derived from the digested food, it nourishes each and every tissue and cell of the body and is analogous to the plasma.
2. Rakta (blood) Dhatu – regarded as the basis of life, it is analogous to the circulating blood cells. It not only nourishes the body tissues, but provides physical strength and colour to the body.
3. Mamsa Dhatu – the muscle tissue. Its main function is to provide physical strength and support for the meda dhatu.
4. Meda (fat) Dhatu – consists of adipose tissue providing support to ashti dhatu. It also lubricates the body.
5. Ashti Dhatu – comprising bone tissues, including cartilage, its main function is to give support to the majja dhatu and the mamsa dhatu.
6. Majja Dhatu – denoting the yellow and red bone marrow tissue, its main function is to fill up the ashti and to oleate the body.
7. Shukra Dhatu – the main aim of this reproductive tissue is to help reproduction and strengthen the body.

Since the dhatus support and derive energy from each other, affecting one can influence others. For instance, interference in the manufacture of the plasma affects the quality of the blood, which in turn affects the muscle. Each tissue type has its own agni which determines metabolic changes in the tissues and forms by-products, which are either used in the body or excreted. Menstrual periods for example are a by-product of rasa. The tissues are also governed by the three doshas, and any imbalance in them also causes imbalances in the dhatus. Heavy periods, therefore, can also be caused by the effects of the excess Kapa on plasma.

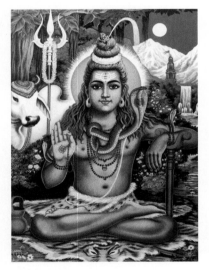

Fig. 2.09 *God Shiva*

Tantra

The word 'Tantra' comes from two Sanskrit words 'tanoti' and 'trayati'. 'Tanoti' means to expand consciousness, and 'trayati' means to liberate consciousness. One might then say that Tantra expands and liberates consciousness, making it the fabric of existence. The highest possible synthesis is between love and meditation. Shiva said of Tantra, 'The truth of the Universe can only be realised within the framework of the physical body.' Simply available as a path to experience full enlightenment.

Yoga

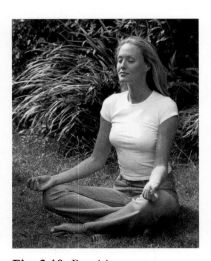

Fig. 2.10 *Practising yoga*

Yoga means 'union with Divine', a philosophy which has to be practised continuously, throughout the day, week, year and life. The ability to be calm in the midst of action, the ability to have a quiet mind in the midst of turmoil is the mark of a true yogi. A lotus (yogi) lives in the marsh (the material world), is unaffected by it but opens its beautiful petals (mind, heart and soul) to the loving grace of the sun (source). The lotus has petals which are unaffected by water (senses/desires) and marsh (ignorance). With its beautiful stem (illumination) it indicates that both can co-exist in the material world, but that without the sun (source), the lotus (yogi) will die. Patanjali, father of Yoga, points out that the liberation and bondage is from one's thoughts.

Such is the inter-dependent matrix between Ayurveda, Yoga and Tantra (Vedic lifestyle) that these three great pillars are the source of perfect health and harmony between mind, body, soul and the environment. The purpose of human life is to attain liberation from the eternal cycle of life and death (Samsara). No attachments to human life are permanent. Therefore liberation through true selfless love for the Divine and all beings is the path to salvation. Hence, every moment which is not spent in the service, love and contemplation of the Divine is wasted. 'For what doth it profit a man, if he gains the whole world, and suffer the loss of his own soul? Or what exchange shall a man give for his soul' (Matthew 16:26 (Bible)).

Most therapists employ an awareness of their belief rather than not knowing the underpinning knowledge that is required to build a healthy, informative understanding. It is the aim of this book to share elementary realisation that makes a healing art of Shiro-Abhyanga a truly holistic application. It is not the purpose of this book to introduce Ayurveda as the only health-care system.

REMEMBER
Yoga means 'union with Divine'.

REMEMBER
Ayurveda means science/knowledge of life.

Key Terms

You need to know what these words mean. Go back through the chapter or check in the glossary to find out.

- Ayurveda
- Tri-Doshas
- Kapa
- Pita
- Vata
- Prakriti
- Tantra
- Yoga
- Srotas
- Tri-Gunas
- Dhatu
- Shiro-Abhyanga
- Satvic
- Rajasic
- Tamasic
- Shiva
- Pantanjali
- Virkurti
- Dhanvantri
- Brahma

3 Introduction to Ayurveda and Bodywork

After working through this chapter you will be able to:

◆ understand the underpinning knowledge of Chakra/Prana/Nadi/Marma Matrix

◆ gain deeper understanding of the multi-dimensional human system

◆ begin to appreciate the spectrun of Ayurveda Bodywork.

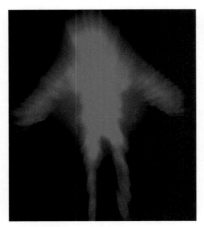

Fig. 3.01 *An aura*

Aura

The subtle anatomy in the multi-dimensional human system is known as the aura – the electromagnetic field. It is ovoid in shape with the widest part around the head and the narrowest under the feet. This multi-dimensional human system is made up of five koshas (or sheaths or energy bodies). Each of these koshas interacts with the others. The layers consist of:

1. Annamaya (the physical body) – food, physical and the five elements.

2. Pranamaya (the etheric body) – breath, vitality and the five primary pranas.
   Closest to the physical body, the first body, lies the etheric body. This second layer is the blueprint for the physical body and disintegrates with it at death. It is in the etheric body where disease starts.

3. Manomaya (the mental body) – impressions, subconscious mind and the five kinds of sensory impressions. It is filled with constantly changing thought forms. Every thought we have creates a form or shape. If we think negative thoughts, they will attract other negative thought forms and thereby amplify the original negativity. The same can also be said of positive thoughts. For this reason, it is most important to be aware of our negativity and endeavour to change it into positive thinking. It is at this level that we are able to get in touch with our intuition. One of life's tasks is to learn to listen to and trust this quiet inner voice. When we are able to tune into our intuition, making the right decisions becomes easier which helps us to walk along our chosen path.

4. Vijnanamaya (the astral body) – ideas, intelligence, directed mental activity. This body contains the record of all our previous lives, plus the reason for our present incarnation. When we reincarnate, we bring with us the knowledge of the path that we have chosen to walk and the challenges we have selected to meet. Unfortunately from the moment of birth, we are subjected to conditioning, which makes us forget our life plan – like leaving the map behind and having to find our way without it.

5. Anandamaya (the spiritual body) – experiences, deeper mind, memory, subliminal and super-conscious mind. The spiritual body is the outer layer of the aura and represents the divine or the true

REMEMBER
The widest part of the aura is found around the head and the narrowest part is found under the feet.

REMEMBER
The etheric body lies closest to the physical body.

REMEMBER
If we think negative thoughts, they will attract other negative thoughts.

self. It is the aspect of each individual, which knows no beginning and no end – the essence of that ultimate reality which we call Goddess, God, Source or Universal Consciousness.

Atma

'Not wounded by weapons, not burned by fire, not dried by wind, not wetted by water, such is the Atma (Soul).' *Bhagwad Gita*

Soul is the ultimate reality; a field of pure potential which expresses itself as conscious energy. The human body is equated to an ashram (healing temple) in which the atma resides.

Karma

Maharishi Patanjali, one of the ancient seers of India, incorporates the law of karma into a time-tested metaphysical science of mind. The Sanskrit word 'karma' means action: mental or physical. It also means the result of action. Past actions, springing from thought waves of desire, cultivate future desires, which in turn result in actions. The law of karma predetermines the soul's future birth; as is one's desire, so is one's destiny. For as is our desire, so is our will; as is our will, so is our deed; and as is our deed, so is our reward, whether good or bad.

Prana

Knowledge of prana is the greatest wisdom – 'Prana vidya maha vidya', *Upanishad*.

There is an old Vedic story about prana that is found in various Upanishads. The five main faculties of our nature – the mind, breath (prana), speech, ear and eye – were arguing with each other as to which one of them was the most important. To resolve this dispute they decided that each would leave the body and see whose absence was most missed.

First, the speech left the body but the body continued, though mute. So the eye left, but the body continued, though blind. Then the ear left, but the body continued, though deaf. And then mind left, but the body continued, though unconscious. Finally the prana began to leave and the body began to die and all the other faculties began to lose their energy.

Prana gives energy to all our faculties, without which they could not function. In India, death is also referred to as the state of a physical being whose pranas (not the soul) have left the body. Yogis and sages participate in elaborate methods of pranayama to retain the pranas in the body, which enhance its longevity.

To bring about positive changes in the body and mind we must understand the energy through which they work. This is called Prana, Chi, Ki, or vital/life-force.

A circular hole is cut in a leaf and then electro-photographed. The image revealed was that of a smaller intact leaf with a tiny hole in it. Examination of the complete amputated leaf reveals a picture of an intact, whole leaf. The amputated portion still appears in the photograph of the leaf even though the missing leaf fragment has been physically removed.

> **REMEMBER**
> The Sanskrit word 'karma' means result of action.

> **REMEMBER**
> Energy is called Prana, Chi, Ki or vital/life-force.

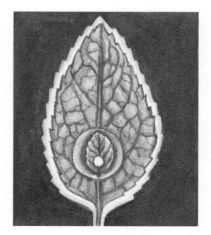

Fig. 3.02 *The phantom-limb phenomenon*

This mirrors the phantom-limb phenomenon which reflects an individual's ability to feel a limb when it has been amputated.

Allopathic (western) doctors have found evidence which suggests that people who have organ transplants can inherit some of their donor's habits. A case was observed where, after receiving a female's heart, a man appeared to change elements of his personality and develop new passions in his life. This, and a number of other cases, have been in the *Journal of Near-Death Studies*.

The flow of prana through the nadis follows bio-rhythmic patterns. The flow of prana through a particular nadi is always highest at a particular time of day or night. Knowledge of this pattern of timing can be helpful in knowing which times to treat a particular Prana and Nadi.

Table 3.01 *Body clock for Prana*

1am – 3am	Liver	3am – 5am	Lungs
5am – 7am	Large intestine	7am – 9am	Stomach
9am – 11am	Spleen/Pancreas	11am – 1pm	Heart
1pm – 3pm	Small intestine	3pm – 5pm	Bladder
5pm – 7pm	Kidney	7pm – 9pm	Heart constrictor
9pm – 11pm	Triple heater	11pm – 1am	Gall bladder

> **REMEMBER**
> Prana empowers the body, mind and soul.

There is nothing in the body that is more subtle than Prana. Even a subtle mental process like thinking can be grasped or reasoned with. Prana is untouchable and unknowable, it empowers the body, mind and soul.

Pranayama

The main method for working on prana is pranayama or Yogic breathing exercises. Yoga emphasises purification of the body (deh) and purification of the mind (citt) as the means to self-realisation. For this reason Ayurveda promotes a karma-free (vegetarian) diet rich in prana or foods full of the life-force, and a mind rooted in ethical values such as honesty and non-violence. Yoga's focal method is purification of the nadis through which the prana flows (Nadishodhana). An impure, toxic or disturbed body and mind cannot realise the higher self.

> **REMEMBER**
> An impure, toxic or disturbed body and mind cannot realise the higher self.

The five primary pranas

The prana matrix divides into five primary types according to movement and direction.

1. **Prana Vayu** – literally the 'forward moving energy' – moves in an inward direction. It governs reception of all types, from the eating of food, drinking of water, and the inhalation of air, to the reception of sensory impressions and mental experiences. It is propulsive in nature, setting things in motion and guiding them. It is located in the head and heart and controls thinking, inhalation, emotions, sensory functioning, memory and receiving cosmic prana from the sun (also known as solar prana). It provides the basic energy that moves us in life. Strong prana is the source of health.

2. **Samana** is the 'equalising or balancing energy' which moves from the periphery to the centre. It is seated in the navel from where it

controls the digestive system and harmonises prana and apana. Samana also governs the digestion of air, emotions and feelings. It is hot and solar in nature. What Samana digests becomes Vyana.

3. **Vyana** is the 'pervading or outward moving energy' as it moves from the centre to the periphery. It is seated in the heart, yet pervades the whole body. It unites the other pranas and the tissues and controls nerve and muscle action. It is responsible for all circulation in the body; food, blood and emotions. Vyana provides strength and stability to the body.

4. **Udana** is the 'upward moving energy' as it moves up the spine to reconnect us to the Divine. It is located in the throat and controls speech, connects us to the solar and lunar forces (sky and earth, masculine and feminine) and is responsible for all spiritual development. Udana controls psychic powers, psychic phenomena and creative expression. The development of the Kundalini relates directly to the Udana prana.

5. **Apana** – literally the 'energy that moves away', it moves downward and outward and governs all forms of elimination and reproduction. On a deeper level it rules the elimination of negative sensory, emotional and mental experiences. It is seated in the colon and controls all the processes of elimination including urine, sweat, menstruation, semen, orgasm, defecation, the foetus, and the elimination of carbon dioxide through breathing. The Apana receives cosmic prana from the earth and the moon. It rules the elimination of negative emotions and provides mental stability. It is also the basis of our immune system and when disturbed is behind the cause of most diseases.

This is much like the working of a machine:

- Prana brings in the fuel (Prana Vayu governs the intake of substances)
- Samana converts this fuel to energy (Samana governs their digestion)
- Vyana circulates the energy to the various work sites (Vyana governs the circulation of nutrients)
- Apana releases waste materials or by-products (Apana governs the elimination of waste materials)
- Udana governs the progressive energy created in the process and determines the work that the machine is able to do (Udana governs the release of constructive energy)

The five secondary Pranas

Table 3.02 *Secondary Pranas and their functions*

Prana	Function
Naga	administers hiccupping
Kurma	administers opening and closing eyes
Krkara	administers digestions
Devadatta	administers yawning
Dhanamjaya	stays after death, still holding the body together

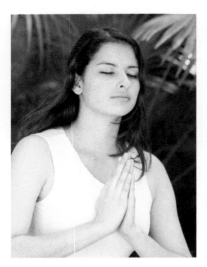

Fig. 3.03 *Meditation accessed through a mantra*

Mantra and meditation

Breathing practices work through pranamaya. However the pranas in the mind can be dealt with directly. Colour and sound (music) are important ways to direct energy in the mind. The best technique is mantra, particularly single syllable or mantras like AUM, which create vibrations (Naad) that can help direct energy into the subconscious. Meditation is accessed through a mantra (spiritual pin code) provided by a guru (remover of ignorance). A mantra is believed to be the sound form of reality, having the power to bring into being the reality it represents.

Studies have suggested that Nam Simran (mantra meditation) is seven times more effective at lowering blood pressure and reducing stress than the customary advice to lose weight and take more exercise. Other benefits of mantra meditation include:

◆ Causes brain wave patterns that demonstrate deep relaxation but with mental alertness
◆ Slows the body's metabolism, heart rate and breathing rate
◆ Raises skin resistance (low skin resistance is related to stress)
◆ Lowers blood pressure
◆ Reduces muscle tension

ACTIVITY

Practise meditating every day.

Nam-simran serves to create more prana in the mind. When the mind is brought to a silent and receptive condition, like the expanse of the sky, a new energy comes into being that brings about great transformations. Ayurveda teaches that meditation and stillness is fundamental for happiness and health. Meditation leads to silence within; it is only in stillness where thought has ceased, that the truth of who we are is revealed. How we meditate is not important, being in it is important. It is through nam-simran that a satvic mind is attained.

Mind

Health by definition is a very holistic concept. The word 'health' comes from the Germanic word meaning wholeness. It was envisaged that you were only healthy when the whole body functioned well. The separation of mind and body is a relatively recent notion. Many non-western countries still treat health and healing according to the wholeness belief system and would consider it foolish to treat a person's physical body without taking into account the state of the mind and soul.

Recent research shows that the brain talks to the body via neuropeptides. The passage of nerve stimulus through the body is well documented, however, research is beginning to show that messages originating from thoughts and emotions are also sent around the body. Studies are beginning to indicate that loneliness can modify the immune system, bereavement may affect the incidence of breast cancer and anxiety alone can increase heart disease. An individual's emotional state will be reflected in the chemical 'soup' that is bathing all our cells, which seems to have a relevance and function in controlling the endocrine, neural and immune systems.

There are many example of the mind/body connection. In athletic pursuits we are aware of the importance of mental rehearsal and de-stressing as a performance enhancer.

The mind/body connection is strongly indicated in the placebo effect. This is when a person responds positively to a physiologically inactive drug such as a sugar pill. Placebos have a remarkably high rate of success – approximately 33% of all cases. If a person believes it will have an effect, it almost invariably does. Evans (1977) found that placebos worked as well as morphine in reducing pain in 50–70% of patients.

The positive reaction is because of the person's belief that the treatment will be effective rather than pain-killing properties of the strategy. The effectiveness of placebos does not indicate that the pain is psychogenic, as 20–40% of people who have had pain induced by a stimulus have reported pain relief with the use of placebos.

Perhaps the most remarkable example of the genius of the body/mind connection is the way in which the physical manifestations of the mind can shift the physiological state in people with split personalities. It is possible for a person with diabetes to find that one personality has low blood sugar levels that need treatment while another, in the same body, may not.

Another example of this was found in a study carried out on an allergic young boy who adopted many different personalities. In one guise he was allergic to orange juice, producing hives on his skin. If another personality emerged the hives would remain, however, the itching would cease immediately and the blisters would begin to subside. This may suggest that the antibodies had a choice of whether to react in the presence of the allergen.

Somewhere there is a decision-making process which allows one aspect of the mind and body to be allergic while another is not. Obviously, much more research is needed in this area but it does illustrate the strong influence that the mind has over the body.

The mind is the gateway to the senses and the bridge between the brain and body. The following four areas are used to adjust and balance the mind.

1. Physical factors
    Diet and lifestyle. Balance the body to help the brain function properly. Consider Vata, Pita and Kapa in equal proportion. Employ Rasayana (rejuvenation) and Panchakarma (purification) therapies together by implementing yoga and pranayama.

2. Psychological factors
    Harmonising the mind and senses promotes a satvic state. Here, the 'right' sensory impressions are offered to the mind as colour (crystal therapy), sound (mantra and chanting), and smell (aromatherapy), as well as meditation and yoga. The intellect must be developed so it can 'digest' these impressions.

3. Social factors
Work, recreation and relationships. The 'right' job, the 'right' companions, the 'right' play. When you can get them 'right' then balance is achieved and good health and contentment is certain.

4. Spiritual factors
Consciousness. The core desire of all consciousness is the attainment of perfect balance and the absolute knowledge of oneself (self-realisation) through mantra-meditation (nam-simran).

The natural state of the mind is satvic. When the mind is calm and clear we perceive truth and have concentration, contentment and devotion. A satvic state is the balance responsible for true health and healing.

Rajasic and tamasic usually work together and cause disease by agitating and deluding, and letting desire, sensory input and emotions overwhelm us. When we have tamasic mind, we become ignorant and deluded. The ego identifies with the physical body and we are dull and limited. Latest research identifies excessive television watching as a factor in poor development of the mind.

Prana and the mind
The mind derives its prana from food and breath.

1. Prana Vayu governs the intake of sensory impressions.
2. Samana governs mental digestion.
3. Vyana governs mental circulation.
4. Udana governs affirmative mental energy, strength and enthusiasm.
5. Apana governs the elimination of toxic ideas and negative emotions.

Determine your mental constitution

ACTIVITY

This basic questionnaire on the opposite page is to determine your state of mind. Add up the number of each quality and give yourself a score.

Ayurveda aims at moving the mind from Tamasic to Rajasic and then to Satvic condition. That is from an ignorant, physical state, to one of vitality and expression, then to peace and enlightenment. A person in a Tamasic state requires Rajasic activity to break up the inertia; a person in Rajasic state requires Satvic activity for calmness. A Satvic person is content and balanced.

	Vegetarian	Some meat	Mostly meat
Diet	☐ Vegetarian	☐ Some meat	☐ Mostly meat
Drugs, stimulants	☐ Never	☐ Occasionally	☐ Frequently
Sensory impression	☐ Calm, pure	☐ Mixed	☐ Disturbed
Sleep	☐ Little	☐ Moderate	☐ Much
Sexual activity	☐ Low	☐ Moderate	☐ High
Control of sense	☐ Good	☐ Moderate	☐ Weak
Speech	☐ Calm	☐ Agitated	☐ Dull
Cleanliness	☐ High	☐ Moderate	☐ Low
Work	☐ Selfless	☐ Personal goals	☐ Lazy
Anger	☐ Rarely	☐ Sometimes	☐ Often
Fear	☐ Rarely	☐ Sometimes	☐ Often
Desire	☐ Little	☐ Some	☐ Much
Pride	☐ Modest	☐ Ego	☐ Vain
Depression	☐ Never	☐ Some	☐ Often
Love	☐ Compassion	☐ Personal	☐ Lacking
Violence	☐ Never	☐ Sometimes	☐ Often
Money	☐ Needs little	☐ Accumulates	☐ Spends all
Contentment	☐ Always	☐ Some	☐ Never
Forgiveness	☐ Forgives	☐ With effort	☐ Grudges
Concentration	☐ Good	☐ Some	☐ None
Memory	☐ Good	☐ Moderate	☐ Poor
Will	☐ Strong	☐ Variable	☐ Weak
Truthfulness	☐ Always	☐ Often	☐ Rarely
Honesty	☐ Always	☐ Sometimes	☐ Rarely
Peace of mind	☐ Generally	☐ Sometimes	☐ Rarely
Creativity	☐ High	☐ Medium	☐ Low
Spiritual study	☐ Daily	☐ Sometimes	☐ Never
Prayer, meditation	☐ Daily	☐ Sometimes	☐ Never
Service	☐ Much	☐ Some	☐ None
Total	**Satvic**	**Rajasic**	**Tamasic**

Table 3.03 *Determine your mental constitution*

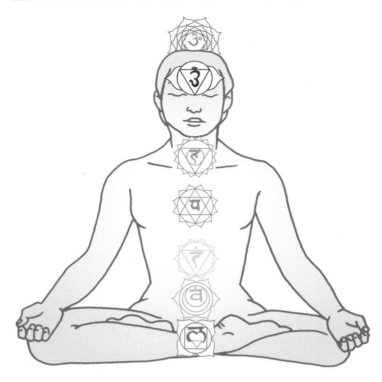

Fig. 3.04 *The 7 primary chakras*

The Sanskrit word 'chakra' means rotation. These unique physic centres are also known as padmas, energy vortex, energy portals or energy gates, which process prana of specific frequencies.

This is a very brief introduction to working of the chakras. In addition to our physical anatomy, there exists a 'subtle' anatomy that is normally unseen. Each chakra corresponds to a different gland and governs specific parts of the physical body and areas of psychological and spiritual development. Assisting these energy centres to remain unblocked is a highly effective way of resisting ill health. Balance between the chakras = vitality and health.

The chakras translate the effects of Pranamaya (the etheric body), Manomaya (the mental body), Vijnanamaya (the astral body) and Anandamaya (the spiritual body) into Annamaya's (the physical body) biological manifestations, via our unique endocrine system.

The endocrine glands are part of a powerful master control system that affects the physiology of the body from the level of cellular gene activation to the functioning of the central nervous system.

The pranamaya network allows Prana of varying vibrational characteristics to flow into the body and influence behaviour at both a cellular and organismic level. In order that incoming subtle energies are properly integrated into the cellular matrix, they must first pass through the four outside bodies.

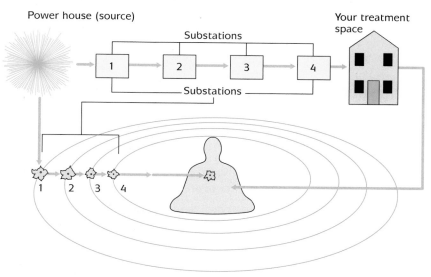

Fig. 3.05 *Step-down transformers*

Once the prana enters through the chakras, it is distributed by a complex network of 72,000 subtle energy channels, or nadis. Modern biological science explains this as the chemical changes produced by the endocrine glands whose secretions mix directly into the body's bloodstream. Nadi network is also known as the meridian system in Chinese/Japanese medical order, and is extensively worked on in acupuncture and shiatsu. Disease is also the result of congestion in the nadi system. It takes the physical body at least two years to manifest that disease. By working on the chakra/nadi/prana/marma system in Indian Head Massage we can achieve a very balanced therapeutic effect.

Ayurveda relates these changes with the five basic tatvas or elements – or doshas. These elements are constantly coming and going with the circadian rhythms inside the body. The ancient Indian science of life, therefore, laid great emphasis on understanding these elements and on working on them accordingly. The chakras are understood to be the playground of the doshas.

Chakra dysfunction may lead to a deprivation of nutritious subtle-energy flow to the body, associated organs and glands supplied by the impaired chakra. If the chakra blockage is chronic, cellular imbalance and disease may eventually occur. Nourishment for the chakras is Hatha Yoga. This form of Yoga is mainly concerned with prana, an expression of which may occur as Asana. Many great Yogis did not learn Asana through mechanical practice but were taught Asana by the power of their awakened prana.

REMEMBER
If the chakra blockage is chronic, cellular imbalance and disease may eventually occur.

Mooladhar

Table 3.04

Yogic name	Prithwi Padma
Meaning of name and essence	Foundation. Mooladhar chakra represents the manifestation of the individual consciousness into human form, that is, physical birth. This chakra encompasses the planes of genesis, illusion, anger, greed and sensuality. The desire for more experience and information acts as a motivating force, a basic impetus for individual development.
Mandala	Four lotus petals encircling a chrome square with a female triangle.
Deity	Bala Brama
Shakti	Dakini
Bija /seed carrier	Elephant Airavata
Position	This chakra located at the base of the spine is the seat of the coiled Kundalini, the vital Shakti. This foundation chakra is the root of all growth and awareness of the divinity of man. In its Yantra form it represents the earth itself.
Tatva/Element	Prithvi (Earth)
Sense	Smell
Gland	Adrenals
Mantra and meditation	Lam. The foundation's root for growth of divinity of man. Beginning of awareness, freedom from disease, inspiration, vitality, vigour, security of inner purity, softness of voice and inner melody.
Primary issue	Survival
Colour	Red. Promotes the sensations of touch, sex, passion, activity, energy, heat and excitement, and reduces fear. Also promotes cheerfulness, enthusiasm, willpower, initiative and courage. Working with this colour will increase psychic ability, mental capacity and fulfil sexual appetite.
Organs governed	Legs, feet, genitals, anus, coccyx and kidneys.
Psychological development	Primordial, origins, survival, sense of grounding, food, shelter, money, rest, exercise, self-care, sense of safety, security
Source of nourishment	Vedic lifestyle including Hatha Yoga
Crystal	Red Tiger's Eye – connects us to our physical self, enhancing the body's health, inner strength, courage and vitality. Tiger's Eye is known for its grounding properties
Healing characteristics	Removes sluggishness and aids in healing depression, anger and sadness. It is useful for activating all under-active conditions of the being (body, mind and soul). Energy boosting and warming.

Svadishthan

Table 3.05

Yogic name	Jal Padma
Meaning of name and essence	Dwelling place of the self. Svadhisthana chakra is dominated by the element of water, the very essence of life. This chakra is the centre of procreation, which is directly related to the moon. Centring on this chakra enables the mind to reflect the world as the moon reflects the sun.
Mandala	Six lotus petals in a circle
Deity	Vishnu
Shakti	Rakini
Bija/seed carrier	Crocodile
Position	Between the navel and genitals
Tatva/Element	Water
Sense	Taste
Gland	Gonads (reproductive glands, ovaries, prostate)
Mantra and meditation	Vam. One acquires the ability to use creative and sustaining energy to elevate oneself in order to refine arts and purify relationships with others, to become free of anger, greed and jealousy. Elevation from the first to the second chakra brings a lunar awareness, reflecting the divine grace of creation and preservation.
Primary issue	Emotions, sexuality
Colour	Orange. The colour promotes sensations of health, confidence and strength, and the use of orange aids the assimilation of new ideas, fellowship, expansion of personal contact and awareness, improves social orientation and fosters exploration and ambition.
Organs governed	Pelvis, genitals, reproductive system, lumbar vertebrae and sacrum.
Psychological development	Vitality, movement, sexual expression, creativity.
Source of nourishment	Vedic lifestyle
Crystal	Carnelian – connects us to our emotional self, enriching intimate feelings and relationships. Helps to remove inhibitions and strengthens our appetite for life!
Healing characteristics	Useful in healing mental disorders: relieves depression, promotes better circulation, reduces anger, aids in ability to focus, improves energy levels, and banishes exhaustion.

Table 3.06

Yogic name	Agni Padma
Meaning of name and essence	Lustrous Gem. Manipur chakra, dominated by the fire element, aids the digestion and absorption of food and thus provides the whole body with the vital energy.
Mandala	Ten lotus petals surrounding a female triangle in a circle.
Deity	Rudra
Shakti	Lakiki
Bija/seed carrier	Ram
Position	The solar plexus, the seat of fire within the body
Tatva/ Element	Fire
Sense	Sight
Gland	Pancreas
Mantra and meditation	Ram. Manipur will bring an understanding of physiology, of internal functioning of the body and of the role of ductless glands in human emotions. The motivation energy of this chakra encourages the person to develop his ego, his identity in the world. The plane of this chakra encompasses karma, good company and selfless service, in the celestial plane. Since the nature of fire is to move upward, when properly tuned Manipur leads the sadhaka in the right direction towards liberation
Primary issue	Self will, personal power
Colour	Yellow. Like red and orange, yellow is a ruling colour and will make other people notice and follow. Yellow promotes the sensation of power, intellect and raw emotion, including change, self-assertion, truth and trust.
Organs governed	Lumbar vertebrae, stomach, gall bladder, liver, diaphragm, nervous system.
Psychological development	Raw emotional energy, desire, ego, personal power, sensitivity.
Source of nourishment	Vedic lifestyle
Crystal	Citrine – connects us to our mental self, improving thought clarity, learning, confidence and self esteem. Helps with mental fatigue and memory.
Healing characteristics	Includes healing digestion, elimination problems, liver dysfunction, intestinal blockages, skin blemishes and stomach pain. Will also aid in curing worry, frustration, pretence, vanity and affectations.

Anahath

Table 3.07

Yogic name	Vayu ma
Meaning of name and essence	Unstuck. Anahath chakra expands in all dimensions and directions as a six-pointed star, air being its tatva, the vital life breath.
Mandala	Hexagram (male and female triangles) encircled by twelve lotus petals.
Deity	Ishana
Shakti	Kakini
Bija/seed carrier	Deer
Position	In the spine at heart level, the seat of balance within the body
Tatva/Element	Air
Sense	Touch
Gland	Thymus
Mantra and meditation	Yam. Once centred in the fourth chakra, one evolves beyond circumstantial and environmental limitations to become independent and self-emanating, gaining wisdom and inner strength.
Primary issue	Love and relationships.
Colour	Emerald. The colour of nature, of the healing that comes through the natural elements. It is the colour of balance and harmony and of our true connection with ourselves. Balancing harmony and nature and to accept the reality that is oneself, all contribute to making green a very helpful stress-relief colour. Emerald is easy on the eye, one of the reasons for its use in operating theatres, and for the green room (the rest rooms) in theatres.
Organs governed	Heart, lungs, chest, breast, thoracic vertebrae, circulatory system.
Psychological development	Love, compassion, service to humanity
Source of nourishment	Vedic lifestyle
Crystal	Aventurine – connects us to unconditional love bringing harmony, forgiveness, sincerity and compassion. Balances our energy, giving a feeling of peace, balance and renewal.
Healing characteristics	It is a useful colour for balancing anything that feels 'intrusive'. Neutralising, soothing, love, compassion, fulfilling. Increases life energy and promotes self-expression, vigour and vitality.

Vishudhi

Table 3.08

Yogic name	Akash Padma
Meaning of name and essence	Pure. Vishudhi chakra is the seat of sound in the body.
Mandala	Sixteen lotus petals surrounding a circle in a crescent.
Deity	Sadashiva
Shakti	Shakini
Bija/seed carrier	Elephant Gaja
Position	Throat
Tatva/Element	Space
Sense	Hearing
Gland	Thyroid
Mantra and meditation	Hum. Here, all elements or tatvas dissolve, becoming pure and self-luminous. Space embodies the essence of all five elements; it is without colour, smell, taste, touch and is form-free of all gross elements. Purification is the vital aspect of this chakra, leading one on the path to divinity, calmness, serenity, purity, and able to read codes in dreams and be in command of mantras. Ability to acquire alternative physical forms.
Primary issues	Communication
Colour	Turquoise. Vibrations are associated with truth, reliability, communication, idealism, transcendental logic and contemplation.
Organs governed	Arms, hands, throat, mouth, voice, lungs, cervical vertebrae, respiratory system
Psychological development	Self-expression, creativity, communication.
Source of nourishment	Vedic lifestyle
Crystal	Sodalite – connects us to the expression of universal truth, reinforcing communication, speech and healing. Ideal for reducing stress and helps to ease the hormonal system.
Healing characteristics	Heals fever, spasms, bleeding, and is calming, cooling, antiseptic and astringent.

Agya

Table 3.09

Yogic name	Guru Padma
Meaning of name and essence	Command. Where true depiction of union of mind, body and spirit takes place. This brings a sense of oneness and unity with the cosmic laws.
Mandala	Oval in shape supported by two lotus petals.
Deity	Hakini
Shakti	Shiva. Half female, half male.
Bija/seed carrier	Sound
Position	Located behind the head, where the spinal cord meets the brain. Western occult science termed this centre of convergence as the 'third eye'.
Tatva/Element	Sound
Sense	Sixth sense
Gland	Pituitary
Mantra and Meditation	Aum. The person evolved through the Agya chakra reveals the divine within and reflects divinity within others. The third eye is the conscious sixth sense revealing the insight of the future. Negative and positive, the components of duality merge, leaving a state of pure grace and neutrality. The mind reaches a state of undifferentiated cosmic awareness. All duality ceases.
Primary issues	Intuitive
Colour	Indigo. Sensations associated include: devotion, intuition, perception and higher vision. Brings self-awareness, telepathy and comprehension.
Organs governed	Forehead, ears, nose, eyes, base of skull, medulla and nervous system
Psychological development	Intuition, intellect, imagination and memories
Source of nourishment	Vedic lifestyle
Crystal	Amethyst – connects us to our unconscious self, heightening our imagination, understanding and intuitiveness. Stimulates dream activity and helps to remove anxieties and fears.
Healing characteristics	Aids neurological diseases.

Table 3.10

Yogic name	Brama Padma
Meaning of name and essence	Thousand-petalled lotus. When one experiences the realms of Sahasrar chakra, one is beyond the conception of the human knowledge. This chakra also allows the entry and exit of the soul.
Mandala	At the centre of a thousand lotus petals is the moon with a female triangle containing Parabindu.
Deity	Par-Brama (total awareness)
Shakti	Maha-shakti (total power)
Bija/seed carrier	Sound
Position	Non-physical crown chakra, Sahasrar is located at the top of the head.
Tatva/Element	Shunya (empty or void), non-existence
Sense	Beyond self
Gland	Pineal
Mantra and meditation	The achievement here is sachianand, truth-being-bliss. The union is achieved with the Source.
Primary Issues	Spirituality
Colour	White. Colour of unity, grace and glory promotes spiritual inspiration, imagination, idealism and superior mentality. White is a combination of all colours and white is no colour. It is everything and nothing. Completeness, emptiness, cleansing, clearing and purifying.
Organs governed	Brain and cerebral cortex
Psychological development	Thinking and decision making
Source of nourishment	Prana
Crystal	Quartz crystal – connects us to our spiritual self, bringing guidance, wisdom and creativity. Purifies our thoughts and feelings, giving us inspiration.
Healing characteristics	Aids in healing aura.

Benefits of working on chakras

Chakra	Level	Action	Prana
Mooladhar	1st	Harmonises	Apana
Svadishthan	2nd	Harmonises	Samana
Manipur	3rd	Calms	Prana Vayu
Anahath	4th	Calms	Vyana
Vishudhi	5th	Harmonises	Udana
Agya and Sahasrar	6th and 7th	Harmonises	Prana Vayu

Table 3.11 *Different Pranas are entertained by different Chakras*

Gems

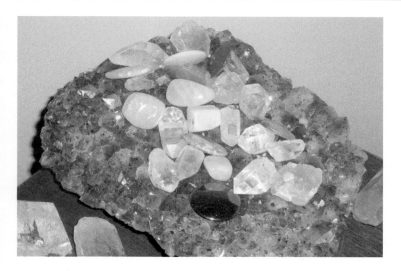

Fig. 3.06 *Selection of gems and crystals*

Gems/crystals have been commonly used in India since the earliest Vedic times, not merely for ornamentation, but for spiritual, occult and healing purposes. They were found to increase the flow of various cosmic energies and used on both individual and collective levels to bring higher forces into life. Jyotish, or science of light, includes astronomy and astrology which are sister therapies to Ayurveda.

Gems are perhaps the most refined form of physical matter. They are something like the flowers of the mineral kingdom. They represent the essence or soul of the earth. According to Vedic astrology, gems represent the concentrated energy of the planets as transmitted to Earth. Gems serve to connect the Earth with the solar system and the stars beyond. Gems are thereby a link between the physical and subtle worlds. Through them it is possible to gain control of the subtle forces of both nature and the psyche.

In India, the best gems were traditionally given to the temples. Gems, as part of the process of worship, serve as a vehicle to bring spiritual forces into the world.

Gems became the basis in ancient cultures, along with mantras, for directing the subtle forces of nature. In this way the Vedic seers were able to direct the energies of fire, water, lightning and the sun.

> **REMEMBER**
> Each type of gemstone has a unique crystalline structure, which vibrates at a particular frequency aiding the flow of prana.

The power of gems on a material level is recognised in modern science and technology, particularly with the use of crystals in computers and lasers. Research continues to determine the subtle power of gems, such as their ability to cure diseases or balance emotions.

There is a new interest in the occult and spiritual use of gems in the West. A number of new systems of gem/crystals usage have arisen. While such approaches are often interesting and creative, they lack a clear foundation.

Colour

Colour is a vibration that we cannot hear but can see. Colours in your environment can affect your chemical balance, causing some strong physical phenomena.

Reds and oranges push increased energy into the adrenal system. In a cascade effect, other related systems may be activated such as the immune, vascular, pulmonary or sexual systems.

Greens and blues soothe and allow the time sense to be accelerated. Time seems to go faster and a wait appears shorter than with a red surrounding. Blues and greens trigger the endocrine system, and a set of neurotransmitters are produced which calm and inspire a slower, gentler spirituality than red.

In the world of work, more and more people are working in artificial light. Businesses around the world enhance their work environment after consultations with colour therapists, to improve working conditions for their employees.

When receiving an Indian Head Massage treatment, the client might visualise a particular colour which is a requirement that the mind and body might be seeking. Suggest wearing, sitting, visualising and eating food of the appropriate colour.

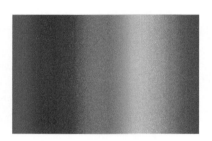

Fig. 3.07 *Colour spectrum*

> **REMEMBER**
> Colour is vibration that we cannot hear but can see.

> **ACTIVITY**
> Visualise a specific colour and think about how that colour makes you feel.

All fruits, vegetables, lentils, seeds and beans are of different colours. It is necessary to cultivate our eating habits by including as much choice of colour as possible in our diet. Drinking water from coloured bottles that have stood in the sun for several hours is a traditional way of taking colour into the body. The water becomes infused with the colour's vibrations and is thus taken directly into the tissues.

The rule with vata is always moderation. Pastel shades of red, orange and yellow are warming, energising and mind clearing. White, blue and green are balancing for pita. Kapa needs rich and warming colours. Red, purple, gold and yellow are best. Shades of blue and green are sedating. Black, brown and grey should be restrained.

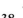

Chakra	Area of the home	Colours	Element
Mooladhar	Entrance hall/stairs	Red/terracotta	Earth
Svadishthan	Dining area	Orange/peach	Earth
Manipur	Living area	Gold/yellow/cream	Fire
Anahath	Kitchen	Emerald/green	Water
Vishudhi	Bedroom	Turquoise/blue	Air
Agya	Study	Indigo/lavender	Air/space
Sahasrar	Meditation/study	White/violet	Space

Table 3.12 *A typical Vastu (holistic concept of architecture and interior design) of an ashram in India*

Sound

Traffic, machines, electrical appliances, radios and television are a major part of our daily lives. Modern noise is so pervasive that unless we take a break away from it, we accept it as normal and become unconscious of the impact it has on us.

Mantras – single or groups of specific syllables – though often associated with spiritual discipline, are also used in Ayurveda for their balancing, nurturing and rejuvenating effect.

For example, Aum – empowers the mind, body and soul and increases Ojas (that which creates a glow of health and beauty). Sanskrit syllables such as relevant mantras assigned to each chakra can be chanted during chakra balancing during an Indian Head Massage session.

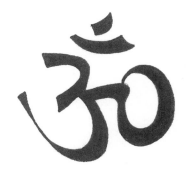

Fig. 3.08 *Aum*

Nadis

The body is the physical component of many interactive energy fields (aura). Each of these fields, or higher dimensional light bodies, is connected to the physical cellular structure through a complex network of energy threads – nadis – through which the prana moves.

Much of the mythology of India is looked at in a very superficial way in the West, when in fact it is filled with much deep, esoteric meaning. Perhaps this is to allow only the capable student to comprehend the real meaning – thus proving their worth as a disciple or sikh.

All nadis originate from the root centre at the base of the spine. There are 72,000 channels which, according to Ayurveda, when blocked to the flow of prana, are the cause of all disease. Of these 72,000 nadis, fourteen are the most important for the massage therapist to recognise.

Fourteen major nadis

Of the fourteen major nadis, there are six on the right side of the body, six on the left side and two in the middle.

Central nadis

1. Sushumna – runs from the base of the spine to the crown. It provides the general upward movement of prana that nourishes the whole body.
2. Alambusha – runs from the beginning of the sushumna to the anus. It provides the outlet for prana to leave the body.

Right nadis

3. Kuhu – runs from the base of the spine up to the second chakra and then to the end of the genitals. Provides prana to the reproductive and urinary tracts.
4. Varuni – runs from the base of the spine up to the fourth chakra and then branches out to provide prana to the whole body.
5. Yashasvati – runs from the base of the spine to the third chakra at the navel, and then branches out to the right arm and right leg. Provides prana to the limbs and allows movement.
6. Pusha – runs from the base of the spine to the sixth chakra at the third eye, and then branches out to provide prana to the right eye.
7. Payasvini – runs from the base of the spine to the sixth chakra at the third eye, and then branches out to provide prana to the right ear.
8. Pingala – runs from the base of the spine to the sixth chakra at the third eye, and then branches out to provide prana to the right nasal passage.

Left nadis

9. Visvodhara –– runs from the base of the spine to the third chakra at the navel and then branches out to provide prana to the abdominal area.
10. Hastijihva – runs from the base of the spine to the third chakra at the navel and then branches out to the left arm and left leg. Provides prana to the limbs and allows movement.
11. Saraswati – runs from the base of the spine to the fifth chakra at the throat, and then branches out to provide prana to the tongue and mouth.
12. Gandhari – runs from the base of the spine to the sixth chakra at the third eye, and then branches out to provide prana to the left eye.
13. Shankhini – runs from the base of the spine to the sixth chakra at the third eye, and then branches out to provide prana to the left ear.
14. Ida – runs from the base of the spine to the sixth chakra at the third eye, and then branches out to provide prana to the left nasal passage.

Shiro-Abhyanga is based on the concept of the release of stagnant prana. The techniques used in the traditional application emanate and augment electrical energy currents in the psychosomatic system. This synchronises the left and right hemispheres of the brain, which has a direct impact on the whole being, leaving the client physically relaxed and mentally serene.

Indian Head Massage regulates the powers of the left side of the body, which has to do with the Ida side of the spine, the lunar cold energy, and connects with the heat of Pingala on the right. With your left hand, work on the left part of the client's body and the right hand on the right side.

Ayurvedic methods work to calm and harmonise the five pranas. This is especially important on the motor organs or sense organs. All the pranas control the nervous system. This awareness is important for anxiety, stress, overwork and other disorders that abuse the senses.

REMEMBER
Ayurvedic methods work to calm and harmonise the pranas.

Ultimately, how much we, as body workers, can help a person through working on the nadis is insignificant compared to the work the client can do themselves. All natural healing comes back to this point – self-responsibility. Any nam-simran or pranayama practice that a person does will benefit him or her. Therefore it is important that we encourage clients to help themselves.

Kundalini

Kundalini is the Sanskrit name given to the energy of the primordial undifferentiated Absolute Consciousness. It is symbolised as a coiled serpent wound around the linga, lying dormant inside the Mooladhar (root chakra) at the base of the spine. Kundalini is the part of the soul which comes and prepares the body before the soul can actually enter it. After the creation of the physical body is completed, it becomes dormant at the base of the spine.

Kundalini, once safely awakened in the prepared individual, expands the limited nature of human consciousness towards a totality of knowledge and experience that climaxes with the ultimate evolutionary consummation, termed self-realisation.

Marma points

Pressure is used on the marmas in the same manner as any other kind of pressure therapy. The marma point is a painful, hard, tender or sensitive point where only gentle pressure should be applied, directed by the client.

As part of Ayurveda, marma massage stimulates the marma points, promoting physical and mental rehabilitation for stroke victims, general weakness, muscle aches/pains and stress. In general, clockwise movements stimulate a marma point, and anti-clockwise movements liberate and dispel blocked or stagnant prana.

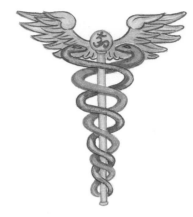

Fig. 3.9 *Kundalini*

> **REMEMBER**
> Kundalini lies dormant inside the Mooladhar (root chakra).

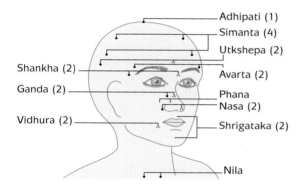

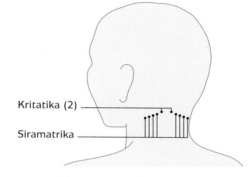

Fig. 3.10 *Nadi junctions*

NB. This illustration depicts the marma points on one side of the head and face only. Corresponding marma points are also represented on the other side.

The key to using pressure therapy on a marma is to work slowly and gently, and to work within the client's comfort zone.

The classic definition of marma in Ayurveda and Yoga is secret. Marma points form a matrix of 108 energy junctions, which stimulate the functions and responses of the body. Marma points are very delicate areas and a hard blow to any of these points may cause extreme trauma. By applying pressure in a systematic way, relief and cure may be given.

Ayurveda believes that the marma points are located at junctions of the body where two major systems meet such as veins and blood vessels, bones and nerves, bones and muscles, ligaments and joints. These nadi junctions are found in the vital areas of the body. The dysfunctioning of any of the marma points may lead to illness.

Massage techniques that address the sensitive marma points should be incorporated during Indian Head Massage. Applying pressure at these points should be done gently, by using the pad of the thumb and fingers. By stimulating marma points one can bring healing effects to a specific

> **REMEMBER**
> The body has 108 marma points.

> **REMEMBER**
> A marma point is found at a nadi junction.

area of the mind-body structure. These points are more importantly used for stimulating internal organs and systems of the body.

Ayurvedic Bodywork modalities

The hallmark of Ayurvedic medicine is that the individual and not the disease is the target of treatment. In contrast to modern medicine, Ayurvedic medicine views disease not as an enemy with which to grapple, but as a manifestation of the breakdown of mechanisms that maintain control, resilience and balance. Dysfunction and disease are rarely organ-specific. Rather, they are an altered systemic physiological malfunction that requires an integrated or holistic model of therapeutic intervention.

Ayurvedic texts warn against giving some of the following listed treatments to those with certain types of contraindications, such as alcoholics, diabetics and pregnant women. This is an exhaustive list for the reader to fully appreciate the spectrum of hands-on modalities within the range of Ayurveda Bodywork.

Abhyanga (body massage)

The concept of Ayurvedic oil massage is entirely different from that of the classical massage techniques, as it balances the tridoshas (Vata, Pita and Kapa) and releases the stored-up stress from the mind and body.

Basti (elimination therapies)

At the end of the treatment each day, after impurities from different parts of the body have been loosened and drawn into the intestinal tract, the client receives a basti. These gentle internal cleansing treatments use either Anuvasana Basti (warm herbalised oil enemas) or Niruha Basti (water-based herbal decoctions) to eliminate impurities from the intestinal tract. This is one of the most important aspects of treatment; Ayurvedic texts say that by basti alone, 50% of illness can be cured.

Chavutti Thirumal (Kalari Uzhichal)

Pronounced cha-vo-te-tie, this massage treatment is a blend of continuously choreographed and rhythmical strokes. Warm oils are used and are administered by the therapist's feet, whilst balancing on one leg and holding onto an overhead pole or rope. Combined with the connected breath-work of the client, there is an overall balancing of all systems, including the nadis and the circulatory systems, a toning and stretching of all muscle tissue, and detoxification of all the major organs.

Garshan

This is a massage with raw silk or wool, which creates friction and static electricity on the surface of the skin and increases circulation in the body. It promotes weight loss and clears away clogging impurities that might cause problems such as cellulite.

Kan Basti (ear treatment)

This remedy improves circulation in the ear, stimulates the brain, lowers blood pressure and helps to balance Vata dosha.

Kati Basti

A special treatment for treating chronic back problems such as a slipped disc, Kati Basti involves immersing the affected areas of the back in lukewarm medicated oil.

> **REMEMBER**
> Abhyanga helps to balance the tri-doshas (Vata, Pita and Kapa).

Kundalini massage

The human spine is a seat of miracles. Ayurveda, Yoga and Tantra, the sciences that deal with the evolution of human consciousness, are full of descriptions of the mysterious Kundalini, the serpent power that lies at the base of the vertebral column. The spine is the seat of seven primary chakras. The arousing of the Kundalini is usually brought about through co-ordination of posture, massage, breath, mantra and a guru.

REMEMBER
The spine is a seat of seven primary chakras.

Marma therapy

Please see Chapter 3, page 41.

Moxibustion (heat treatments)

Heat treatments dilate the srotas (the channels of the body such as the arteries, veins and lymph system) allowing the impurities that were loosened through oil massage to be swept away. Heat helps loosen the impurities (ama) so they can be broken down and eliminated more easily. The ama becomes less solid and begins flowing toward the intestinal tract for elimination.

Nasya therapy (herbal inhalation therapy)

This treatment purifies the head and energises all the senses. Nasya helps to remove microcytic elements with the application of medicated oils into the nasal passage. This stimulates the nerves and tissues, and provides relief from migraines, sinusitis, chronic colds and chest congestion, and induces sound sleep.

Netra Basti (eye treatments)

A treatment which helps to remove impurities from the eyes, and includes ghee eyebaths and herbal smoke treatments to cleanse these important organs.

Nuh therapy (nail diagnosis)

White spots on nails show calcium and zinc deficiency. Bitten nails show nervousness and mineral deficiency. Brittle nails show low iron or vitamin A. Split nails show low Agni in the stomach. Yellowish nails show a liver imbalance. Bluish nails show lung and heart imbalance. Pale nails show poor blood circulation   or anaemia.

Padam-Abhyanga (reflexology)

Foot massage before going to sleep is highly praised in Ayurveda. The art of reflexology states that specific points on the feet and hands mirror various organs of the body, which may be stimulated by foot/hand massage.

REMEMBER
Reflexology involves treating specific points on the feet and hands that mirror various organs of the body.

Pancha Karma

Pancha Karma treatments are the anchor of Ayurveda. A purification therapy is designed to assist the body in the internal cleansing process by eliminating the toxins, wastes and other excesses to bring the supportive forces of life and the tridoshas into balance. Pancha Karma includes five procedures:

1. Vamana (therapeutic vomiting)
2. Virechana, Vireka (purgation therapies)
3. Basti

4. Nasya
5. Rakta Mokshana (blood letting)

There is set of preliminary treatments called Purva Karma given prior to Pancha Karma. These are:

- Sneha – herbal oil application (external, oral, rectal)
- Swedana – herbal diaphoretic therapy (steam bath)
- Shirodhara – special oil stream for the third eye

REMEMBER
Pinda Swedana involves a paste made from herbs and grains boiled in milk that is rubbed onto the body.

Pinda Swedana

A medicated paste of herbs and grains boiled in milk is made into a poultice and rubbed onto the whole body in a synchronised pattern. The treatment revitalises the body by imparting nourishment to the tissues, restores energy and mobility, and relieves stress.

Pizichill

This is a massage technique that protects from illness and builds up immunity for a healthy life. It gives a multitude of relief from the easing of rheumatic or joint pains, to strengthening the muscles, nerves and tissues, and slowing the ageing process. The massage is carried out through a constant flow of hot, herbal oil.

Shiro Basti

Warm herbal medicated oil is held for about one hour within a closely fitted cap around the head, thus allowing the scalp to soak in the therapeutic oil. This treatment is highly effective for headaches and migraines, insomnia, dryness of the nose, eyes and mouth. Also useful for memory loss, mental stress and strain, vata vitiation as well as vata diseases, back and spine problems, sinusitis, chronic colds, facial paralysis and hallucinations. This is one of Ayurveda's important external oleation methods.

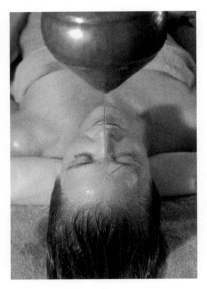

Fig. 3.11 *Shirodhara*

Shirodhara

A stream of special oil is poured over the forehead, balancing vata dosha and vata disorders such as insomnia, anxiety or worry. Shirodhara is a cooling treatment that settles the mind and profoundly relaxes the central nervous system. It is specifically said to strengthen the dhatus, to nourish the nervous system, to increase the glow of the complexion, to increase stability in the mind and to remove malaise.

REMEMBER
Shirodhara involves pouring special oil over the third eye.

Shirolepa

The head and shoulders are given a mild massage after which a medicated paste is applied on the head. This stabilises the nervous system and activates the marma points in the scalp and head offering a unique soothing effect to the whole body.

Swedana (sweat treatments)

Sitting on a stool, the client's body is enclosed in a wooden cabinet and surrounded by a therapeutic application of heat. The pores and channels of the body open in order to release ama (toxins). The head is not enclosed and is protected from the heat. The vapours soften and dilate the channels of the body, allowing the impurities to pass out. It is particularly beneficial for musculo-skeletal problems, earache, headache, asthma, coughs and many other disorders.

Vajikaran (virilification therapy)

This produces longer and better sexual performance.

Vishesh

This massage is for deep-seated muscle aches and pains and for removing stubborn toxins.

Uzhichil

This full body massage is effective in enhancing blood circulation, alleviating pain and relieving tense nerves and muscles, thus relaxing the body.

Udvartana

This herb-based paste massage improves peripheral circulation, thereby improving complexion.

Progress Check

1. What are the layers that make up the aura?
2. What are the five primary pranas?
3. What is meant by nadis?
4. What is marma massage?
5. Briefly describe Abhyanga.

Key Terms

You need to know what these words mean. Go back through the chapter or check in the glossary to find out.

- Atma
- Annamaya
- Pranamaya
- Manomaya
- Vijnanamaya
- Anandamaya
- Karma
- Prana
- Pranayama
- Prana Vayu
- Samana
- Vyana
- Udana
- Apana
- Meditation
- Chakras
- Nadis
- Kundalini
- Marma points
- Abhyanga

Anatomy and Physiology Systems

After working through this chapter you will be able to:

◆ understand the structure and function of all 11 body systems

◆ recognise the effects of massage on these systems.

At Ayurveda's core is the belief that people are a combination of mind (manh), body (dey) and soul (atma) within the universal context, and that those who live in harmony with nature and their inner being are healthy. Massage is nourishing, it pacifies vata and kapa, relieves fatigue, provides stamina, pleasure and quality sleep, enhances the complexion and the lustre of the skin, promotes longevity, and nourishes all parts of the body. Better, deeper sleep at night increases levels of stamina through the day. Massage reduces muscle tension and relieves pain and opens the pores.

There is no excuse for undermining the health of the human body, the most wondrous creation of the Supreme Divine. Perfect in every detail, with working parts that replace themselves constantly, built-in thermostats to guard against the cold and changes in the atmosphere, an automatic cooling system that refreshes you in the extreme heat and essential organs that work for twenty-four hours every day and never go on strike, unless you overload them, and do their particular jobs to the very best of their ability.

No engineer could ever design a machine that could do the same job over and over again throughout such a long period of time; no heating expert has ever devised such a marvellous automatic system. Look at the wonderful way everything within this physical structure, called the human body, can not only look after itself and arrange its own maintenance, but also renew its own parts.

It has within itself a huge workforce, which it feeds, houses and replaces at very short notice. It has the most efficient power and sewerage systems ever designed. This is a wonder of wonders, a miracle of miracles, a treasure beyond all treasures, and yet many constantly abuse it every day. Sending the workers on strike, killing off the army of protectors, severely overloading the power and sewerage systems and packing out the warehouses with useless rubbish so that there is no space left for essentials. If you owned the greatest treasure in the world, how would you look after it?

You would make sure that it was fully protected in every possible way; you would see that it was kept at the right temperature and regularly cleaned so that its beauty could be admired by everyone and you would be proud to put it on show for the whole world to see.

How is the body made up?

We think first of the major organs – the heart, the brain, the liver, the lungs; and then perhaps the arms and legs and other parts. When we are thinking of health, however, we need to look at something much smaller – the cells of the body. In our bodies there are millions and millions of them. They are minute and can only be seen under a microscope. Our total health is determined by the health of our cells. For all our life they are living units that breathe, feed and excrete, reproduce and die.

Each cell is like a tiny city. It has a wall called a membrane. The inside of the city is filled with a fluid called cytoplasm. It is essential for this fluid to be of the right chemical balance. Our bodies are made up of about 65% water; some is in the cells and some is in the tiny spaces between. The fluid on the inside of the cell has to have potassium to work well, while the water outside has to have sodium. If these get out of balance through a less than healthy lifestyle, the cell cannot work so well. This balance should be maintained by what we eat and drink day to day.

Inside the cell city itself are several round structures called ribosomes. These are where the building materials – protein – are made. There are other factories which make the building materials for the construction of the body. These are the golgi apparatus and the endoplasmic reticulum.

The different factories need to have energy to run them, and this comes from the power stations called the mitochondria. Other workers in our cells are called lysosomes. Their task is to bring in the food and then, when each factory in the city has had enough, they take up the leftovers, eating it to recycle it.

The city has a town hall too, called the nucleus where the decisions are made, as to whether to make new cells just like itself, or what colour they will be and what shape and size.

All these billions of cells throughout you are waiting every day to see what foods you will put into your mouth to feed them. They do their best with the sugars and the fats and the heavy proteins they receive, but they are very happy when you give them lots of fresh fruit for the potassium they need, and lighter, less clogging, natural foods – grains, fruit, vegetables, beans, nuts and seeds. There is electricity in the cells too, which is more active when the cells have plenty of oxygen. They then energise the brain and the muscles. Eating raw fruits and vegetables give the best results. If you have too much fat the cells are starved of oxygen and will eventually give up their struggle. They need a clean environment in which to thrive and do their work. Large amounts of protein create more waste than the body can cope with and results in disease. We need foods that work with the body and keep it in balance.

So remember that inside you are billions of little living things all waiting to see what you will give them today. They depend on you. If you feed them well they will give you better health and increased energy in return, your skin will look better, your eyes brighter and you will have improved thinking power and more physical stamina to cope with life.

> **REMEMBER**
> Our bodies contain millions and millions of cells.

> **REMEMBER**
> The body is made up of 65% water.

> **REMEMBER**
> When your cells are truly 'alive' many health problems will be reduced and you will feel leaner and more awake.

If cells are not fed properly, a sticky sludge develops between them and they live in a swamp with little oxygen and lots of toxins. Bacteria grow there too. It is no surprise then, that we feel unwell some days! When we are ill, the electrical activity in the cells decreases which means they do not reproduce so readily. It is only their reproduction that makes healthy growth and development in children possible or the repairs needed in adult bodies.

The answer – give your body a spring clean and then make a fresh start. The amazingly optimistic thing is that cells soon respond and begin to function better. In three weeks' time many will have reproduced and you can treat these new ones with proper care, in a new healthy way.

A good knowledge of human anatomy and physiology is the hallmark of a good Indian Head Massage practitioner.

Anatomy and physiology

The anatomy and physiology contained in this book is endorsed by the Ayurvedic Bodywork Consortium as it places significant emphasis on the basic understanding of anatomy and physiology. It is essential to recognise the basic importance of the human structure and function.

- Anatomy is the study of the structure and the relationship among structures
- Physiology is the study of how body structures function

Homeostasis

Homeostasis (homeo=same, stasis=standing still) is a state in which the body's internal environment remains within certain physiological limits in terms of chemical composition, temperature and volume. All body systems attempt to maintain homeostasis.

> **REMEMBER**
> The imbalance of homeostasis leads to weakness leading to demise.

The human body is made up of eleven systems which are outlined below with their major components and functions. All systems address the organisation, support, movement, integration, control, regulation, maintenance, reproduction and development of the being.

The study of anatomy and physiology is based on the assumption that the body works perfectly, but in reality this is rare. Therefore we have to study the abnormalities, illnesses of structure and function and drug regimes which come into professional consideration when offering treatments.

An overview on all of the eleven systems
Cardiovascular system
Heart, blood vessels and blood transport nutrients, waste products, gases and hormones throughout the body. It plays a role in the immune response and the regulation of body temperature.

Digestive system
Mouth, oesophagus, stomach, intestines and the accessory structures. It performs the mechanical and chemical processes of digestion, absorption of nutrients and elimination of wastes.

Endocrine system

Endocrine glands – pineal, pituitary, thyroid, parathyroid, thymus, adrenal (suprarenal) glands, pancreatic islets (islets of langerhans), ovaries/testes. A major system which controls the regulation of metabolism, reproduction and many other functions.

Integumentary system

Skin, hair, nails and sweat glands. Protects, regulates temperature, prevents water loss and produces vitamin D precursors.

Lymphatic system

Lymph vessels, lymph nodes and other lymph organs. The system removes foreign substances from the blood and lymph, combats disease, maintains tissue fluid balance and absorbs fats.

Muscular system

Muscles attached to the skeleton allow body movement, maintain posture and produce body heat.

Nervous system

Brain, spinal cord, nerves and sensory receptors. A major regulatory system which detects sensation, controls movement and physiological and intellectual functions.

Reproductive system

Gonads, accessory structures and genitals perform the process of reproduction and control sexual functions and behaviours.

Respiratory system

Lungs and respiratory passages exchange gases (oxygen and carbon dioxide) between the blood and the air, and regulate blood pH.

Skeletal system

Bones, associated cartilage and joints. The system protects and supports, allows body movement, produces blood cells and stores minerals.

Urinary system

Kidneys, bladder and ducts that carry urine. This system removes waste products from the circulatory system: regulates blood pH, iron balance and water balance.

The cardiovascular system

Structure of blood

Blood is made up of 55% plasma, which surrounds the cells, and 45% of various types of cell.

Red blood cells

Red blood cells are made in the bone marrow. When fully formed the nucleus disappears. The cells contain haemoglobin (red pigment) which is involved in the transport of oxygen around the body. Red blood cells are very small, thus providing a large surface area over which oxygen can be absorbed. The cells only live for about 120 days, after which they are broken down by the liver and the iron from the haemoglobin is recycled.

White blood cells

White blood cells are concerned with the body's defences. These largest of the blood cells have no haemoglobin. They contain a nucleus and some have granules in their cytoplasm. There are fewer white blood cells than red, approximately one white cell to every 600 red cells. There are two types of white blood cell:

1. Phagocytes form about 75% of white blood cells. They seek out harmful micro-organisms and ingest and destroy them.
2. Lymphocytes form about 25% of white blood cells; they do not ingest bacteria, but form antibodies to protect the body against infection.

Platelets

Platelets are minute round discs which disintegrate rapidly when blood is shed to aid blood clotting. There are approximately 300,000 platelets per cubic millimetre of blood. The platelets are made in the bone marrow. Plasma is a straw-coloured, transparent liquid in which different types of cells are suspended.

Functions of the blood

The blood has two main functions:

1. Defence – defending the body against infection. This occurs in three main ways:

   a) Phagocytosis – phagocytes engulf foreign material in the blood, or they may squeeze through the capillary walls to reach infection in the tissues. Pus is a yellow substance consisting of dead phagocytes and bacteria and is a sign that the body is fighting infection.
   b) Immune response – antibodies are produced by the lymphatic system. The antibodies become attached to the microbe and destroy it.
   c) Clotting – if platelets are damaged, a process is initiated from which a stringy substance called fibrin is produced. Fibrin forms a network, which entangles red blood cells to form a clot. The clot dries to form a scab which prevents further loss of blood, prevents entry of bacteria, and protects new tissues as they develop.

2. Transports – blood transports food, oxygen, waste products and hormones around the body, and white blood cells to areas of infection.

   a) Oxygen is carried from the lungs to the body cells. Haemoglobin in the red blood cells picks up the oxygen and become oxyhaemoglobin. When it reaches the cells it gives up the oxygen and becomes haemoglobin again.
   b) Carbon dioxide from the body cells is dissolved in the plasma, and carried to the lungs where it can be breathed out.
   c) Digested food, e.g. glucose and amino acids, is carried from the small intestine to the liver, and then travels around the body in the plasma.

d) Hormones are carried in the plasma, from the endocrine glands to target organs.
e) Urea is carried in the plasma from the liver, where it is made, to the kidneys, where it is then excreted in the urine.
f) Heat is carried by all parts of the blood, from the liver and muscles, to all parts of the body.

Circulatory system

The circulatory system consists of the heart which acts as a pump and a continuous network of blood vessels through which the blood circulates. Blood is carried away from the heart in the arteries and back to the heart through the veins.

Arteries

- Carry blood away from the heart
- Carry oxygenated blood (except the pulmonary artery)
- Have thick muscular walls, which prevent them from bursting under the pressure of the blood
- Have a small lumen
- Carry blood at high pressure
- Have no valves (except in the walls of the main arteries leaving the heart)
- Divide to form smaller arterioles

Veins

- Carry blood towards the heart
- Carry deoxygenated blood (except the pulmonary vein)
- Have thin walls with a thin muscular layer
- Have a large lumen
- Carry blood at low pressure
- Have valves which lie flat when blood flows in the correct direction and close to prevent blood flowing backwards
- Subdivide into smaller venules

Capillaries

- Minute vessels that are formed when the arterioles divide
- Walls consist of a single layer of cells which allow substances to diffuse across easily
- Are found in every part of the body forming a network
- Join to form venules

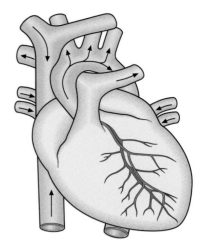

Fig. 4.01 *The heart*

REMEMBER
The smallest vessels are called capillaries, arterioles and venules.

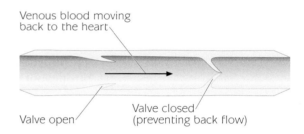

Venous blood moving back to the heart

Valve open   Valve closed (preventing back flow)

Fig. 4.02 *A valve in a vein*

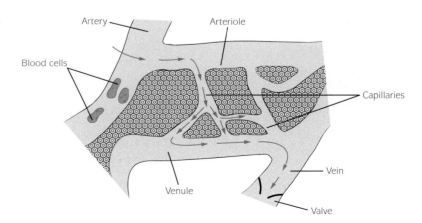

Artery   Arteriole

Blood cells

Capillaries

Venule

Vein

Valve

Fig. 4.03 *How blood passes from arteries through capillaries to veins*

Heart

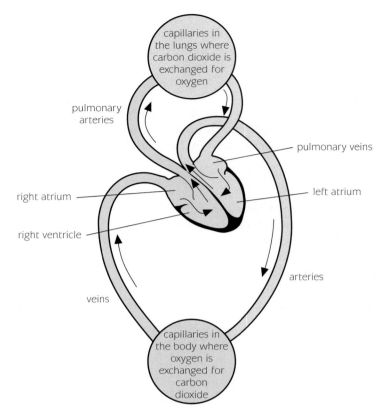

capillaries in the lungs where carbon dioxide is exchanged for oxygen

pulmonary arteries

pulmonary veins

right atrium

left atrium

right ventricle

arteries

veins

capillaries in the body where oxygen is exchanged for carbon dioxide

Fig. 4.04 *The heart and cardiovascular system*

The function of the heart is to maintain the circulation of blood throughout the body.

Structure
- A roughly cone-shaped, hollow, muscular organ
- Approximately 10 cm long, the size of a clenched fist
- Weighs about 225 g

The walls of the heart consist of three layers of tissue:

1. Pericardium – is made up of two sacs: the outer sac includes fibrous tissue which prevents over-distension of the heart, the inner sac contains serousmembrane, which secretes fluid to allow smooth movements when the heart beats.
2. Myocardium – is composed of cardiac muscle which is only found in the heart.
3. Endocardium – is a thin, glistening membrane which forms a lining to the myocardium.

The heart is divided into a right and left side by a wall called the septum. Each side is divided again by valves into an upper chamber called the atrium and a lower chamber called the ventricle.

> **REMEMBER**
> The human heart is described as a double pump because the right and left sides are separate but pump together.

Summary

- Blood passes from the right side of the heart to the left side via the lungs.
- Both atria contract followed by the simultaneous contraction of both ventricles
- The right side deals with deoxygenated blood
- The left side deals with oxygenated blood

Pulse

The pulse is described as a wave of distension and elongation felt in the artery wall. It is caused by the contraction of the left ventricle which forces about 60 to 80ml of blood into the already full aorta. When the aorta is distended, a wave passes along the walls of the arteries. This can be felt at any point where an artery can be pressed gently against a bone. The number of pulse beats per minute varies considerably in different people and in the same person at different times. An average of 60 to 80 beats per minute is common.

Factors affecting the pulse rate

There are a number of factors which can affect an individual's pulse rate. These include:

Position – when the individual is standing up the pulse rate is usually more rapid than when lying down.
Age – pulse rate in children is more rapid than in adults.
Sex – men have a more rapid pulse than women.
Exercise – any exercise will increase the pulse rate. The resting pulse should be restored soon after exercise has stopped.
Emotion – the pulse rate is increased due to strong emotional states, e.g. excitement, fear, anger or grief.

ACTIVITY

Feel the pulse in your wrist and then take some exercise and feel the pulse again. The heart rate is faster so the pulse rate will be faster.

Effects of massage on blood circulation

Slight pressure applied by effleurage strokes along the arms, legs, chest and back aids the movement of blood from the extremities back to the heart. Firmer pressure applied by petrissage strokes brings a rapid increase of fresh blood to the area it is being applied to. The increased movement of blood carries waste products, toxins and carbon dioxide away from the area. In return, fresh blood flows into the area which improves its metabolism as the food supply to the area is enhanced.

The physiological and psychological effects of massage on the cardiovascular system

- Improves blood circulation (taking the pressure off the arteries and veins).
- Reduces oedema, adhesions in tissues after injury, and muscular spasm, improves muscle tone and eliminates waste.
- Increased circulation, especially to nerve endings.

- Strengthens the heartbeat. When the rate of heartbeat decreases, high blood pressure may be reduced.
- Warmth is produced in the area due to increased blood flow and friction of the hands of the therapist.
- May reduce viscosity of the blood, therefore reducing its rate of coagulation.

The digestive system

The alimentary canal is a long tube through which food passes. It consists of the following structures: mouth, pharynx, oesophagus, stomach, small intestine, large intestine, rectum and anal canal. A number of accessory organs are involved in the digestive process, helping to break down toxins and other waste matter that digestion produces. They include the teeth, tongue, salivary glands, gall bladder, pancreas and liver.

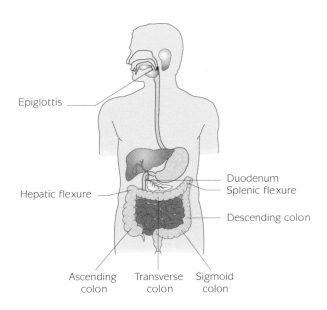

Fig. 4.05 *The digestive system*

The digestive process is a combination of several chemical reactions that act on the food we eat. Food is composed of fats, carbohydrates (or starches) and proteins. These are broken down into their relative chemical compounds so that the body can use them.

Digestion is the breakdown and transformation of solid and liquid food into microscopic substances. There are five stages of activity:

1. Ingestion – the process of taking food into the alimentary tract
2. Propulsion – the process of moving the contents along the alimentary tract
3. Digestion – the mechanical breakdown of food by mastication (chewing), the chemical digestion of food by enzymes secreted by glands and accessory organs of the digestive system
4. Absorption – the process by which digested food substances pass through the walls of some organs of the alimentary canal, into the blood and lymph capillaries for circulation around the body
5. Elimination – the process of excreting food substances, which cannot be digested or absorbed by the bowel, as faeces

> **REMEMBER**
> Substances are moved along the digestive tract by a series of muscle contractions known as peristalsis.

Metabolism is the process by which the body converts food and other substances into energy to be used for growth, repair and maintenance of a fit and healthy body. Part of this process is the digestion of food which when broken down is absorbed and used in the metabolic process, providing energy. Incorrect metabolism can cause minor health problems, such as sluggish skin, excess weight and greasy or spotty skin. Massage can help to stimulate metabolism and improve the general health of the body.

The physiological and psychological effects of massage on the digestive system

- Aids the function of the digestive organs.
- Helps with the release of enzymes and breakdown of food to eliminate poisons from the body through sweat.
- It stimulates the digestive system and activates the urinary system.
- Promotes peristaltic activity in the colon (enhancing the elimination of faecal matter and combating constipation and flatulence).
- As well as helping the digestion and elimination of food, massage also increases the absorption of digested foods (nutrients).

The endocrine system

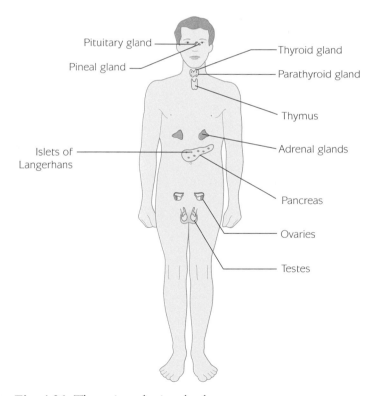

Fig. 4.06 *The main endocrine glands*

The endocrine system is one of the body's communication systems. It works with the nervous system to co-ordinate the body's activities. It consists of the endocrine glands and the hormones or chemical messengers they secrete and/or store. Hormones affect the behaviour and function of the different areas of the body. For example, hormones are responsible for the rate of growth, changes during puberty, the menstrual cycle, pregnancy, the menopause, responses to stress and danger, as well as the correct function of the kidneys and the digestive system.

An endocrine gland is a ductless gland, which produces hormones. Ductless means there is no separate canal or tube to transport the hormones into the bloodstream. The secretory cells of the endocrine gland cluster around blood capillaries inside the gland, so the hormones can readily pass into the blood. There they become attached to plasma proteins and are transported to the target organ, or organs, in which they produce a response.

> **REMEMBER**
> A hormone is a chemical messenger.

A hormone is a chemical messenger that is secreted directly into the blood by a particular gland. Some hormones are made of protein (like insulin), others are steroids (adreno-corticoid hormones), glycoproteins (FSH, LH, TSH) and derivates of amino acids.

The endocrine system consists of a number of distinct glands and some tissue in other organs. Although the hypothalamus is part of the brain and not an endocrine gland as such, it controls the pituitary gland and has an indirect effect on many other glands. The endocrine glands are:

One pituitary gland
Situated at the base of the brain, the pituitary gland is closely connected to the hypothalamus. It has two hormone-secreting lobes, the anterior and posterior lobes.

Anterior pituitary lobe
The anterior pituitary lobe secretes the following hormones:

- Human growth hormone (HGH)
  Regulates growth and height. Hypersecretion causes gigantism or acromegaly; hyposecretion causes dwarfism.

- Melanocyte stimulating hormone (MSH)
  Stimulates the production of melanin in the skin.

- Thyrotrophin (TSH)
  Contols the thyroid gland.

- Adrenocorticotrophin (ACTH)
  Controls the adrenal cortex.

- Prolactin or lactogenic hormone (LTH)
  Produces milk during lactation.

- Gonadotrophins (gonad/sex organ hormones)
  Control sexual development and related organs.

- Follicle stimulating hormone (FSH)
  Stimulate ovaries to produce oestrogen and to ovulate in women; stimulates sperm production in men.

- Luteinising hormone (LH)
  Stimulates ovaries to produce the corpus luteum from ruptured follicles, and to produce progesterone.

- Interstitial cell stimulating hormone (ICSH) / luteinising hormome in men
  Stimulates sperm production and secretion of testosterone.

Posterior pituitary lobe

The posterior pituitary lobe secretes the following hormones:

- Antidiuretic hormone (ADH or vasopression)
  Regulates water absorption into the kidneys. Hyposecretion causes diabetes insipidus, hypersecretion causes oedema (swelling).

- Oxytocin
  Contracts mammary glands during suckling, releases milk secreted into ducts, contracts uterus muscles during childbirth.

One thyroid gland

- Situated in the neck
- Hormones produced are: thyroxin, triiodothryronine and calcitonin produced in response to TSH
- Stimulates tissue metabolism, maintains basic metabolic rate (BMR)
- Hypersecretion can lead to Graves' disease or thyrotoxicosis, hyposecretion can cause body systems to slow below normal speed, cretinism (at birth), or myxoedema (a disorder caused later in life by untreated cretinism)
- Maintains calcium and phosphorus balance

Four parathyroid glands

- Four glands, two at either side behind the thyroid
- Produces parathormone
- Maintains calcium levels in plasma, stimulates calcium re-absorption in kidneys, activates vitamin D
- Hypersecretion can lead to softened bones and spontaneous bone fractures, hyposecretion can lead to abnormally low calcium levels, tetany and convulsions

Two adrenal (suprarenal) glands

Situated on top of each kidney, they are split into two parts, the adrenal cortex and the adrenal medulla.

Adrenal cortex

The adrenal cortex secretes:

Mineralcorticoids – aldesterone (steroids)

- Regulate body salts, especially sodium chloride and potassium
- Hypersecretion: kidney failure, high blood pressure, abnormal heartbeat due to increased levels of potassium in the blood; hyposecretion: Addison's disease, muscular atrophy and weakness, slow down of body systems

Glucocorticoids (steroids)

- Produced in response to ACTH, metabolises carbohydrates, fats and proteins
- Malfunctions can lead to stunted growth, Cushing's syndrome, hypertension, moon-shaped face, muscular atrophy and diabetes mellitus

Sex hormones (steroids)

- Female – oestrogen and progesterone
- Male – testosterone
- Aids sexual development and maturity, ovulation; hair growth in pubic and axillary areas

> **REMEMBER**
> The pituitary gland is known as the master gland because it controls many other glands.

- Malfunctions can lead to many disorders including hirsutism, amenorrhoea and Addison's disease

Adrenal medulla
- Supports the nervous system
- Adrenaline and noradrenaline – also known as stress hormones, they prepare the body for fight or flight by speeding up the heart rate, slowing digestive and urinary systems, increasing blood pressure and blood sugar levels, increasing metabolic rate and dilating the pupils. Adrenaline is an important vasoconstrictor as it constricts blood vessels in order to increase blood pressure

The pancreatic islets (islets of Langerhans)
- Situated behind and slightly below the stomach between the duodenum and spleen
- Produce insulin and glucagon
- Helps glucose enter cells, thus regulating blood sugar levels
- Hyposecretion can cause diabetes mellitus, fatigue, weight loss, coma, hypersecretion can lead to hypoglycaemia (low blood sugar level) including symptoms of hunger and sweating

Two ovaries (in females)
Situated either side of the uterus, the ovaries produce the female sex hormones oestrogen and progesterone (the testes also produce a small amount in men).

- Responsible for female characteristics, e.g. breast growth, widening of hips, pubic and axillary hair growth
- Hyposecretion of luteinising hormone can lead to polycystic ovarian syndrome (PCOS), hypersecretion of oestrogen in males can lead to muscle atrophy and breast growth

Two testes (in males)
Situated within the scrotum behind the penis, the testes produce the male sex hormone testosterone (the ovaries also produce a small amount in women).

- Responsible for male characteristics, e.g. sperm production, changes at puberty – voice breaking, pubic, facial and axillary hair growth, increased muscle mass
- Hypersecretion can lead to virilism, hirsutism and amenorrhea

One pineal gland (or pineal body)
Situated in the centre of the brain, the pineal gland produces melatonin.

- Controls body rhythms, responds to sunlight
- Malfunctions can lead to feelings of being jet-lagged, depression, seasonal affective disorder (SAD)

One thymus gland
Situated in the thorax, the thymus gland produces thyroid hormones.

- Strengthens the immune system
- Malfunction can lead to lowered immunity and/or stress, Grave's disease and thyroiditis

The physiological and psychological effects of massage on the endocrine system

Hyperthyroidism is a condition in the endocrine system in which the thyroid glands produce excessive amounts of thyroxine. Massage may be favourable to the client to help treat this as it helps to carry hormones to the blood's plasma.

Hypoglycemia, another condition in the endocrine system, is a result of having inadequate amounts of glucose in the blood. This may be caused by stress, infection or under-eating. After consuming fruit juice, massage may be offered, when the symptoms have settled.

Hypothyroidism is a condition in which circulating levels of thyroid hormones are unusually low. Massage may be a supportive contribution.

Metabolic syndrome (or insuline resistance syndrome) is a collection of symptoms that indicate a high risk of several diseases such as atherosclerosis, diabetes, and even a stroke or heart attack. If the client can make adjustments to his or her diet and exercise programme, massage can be appropriate.

The integumentary system

Skin

The skin has the largest surface area of any organ in the body, and is the heaviest. On the surface are the sensitive papillae, and within are certain structures with special functions: the sweat glands, hair follicles and sebaceous glands. The skin protects the internal organs of the body against infection, injury and harmful sunrays. It also plays an important role in the regulation of body temperature.

Although the skin of an average-sized adult may weigh as much as twenty pounds, it is only paper-thin in some places. The skin is composed of two tissues, an outer layer called the epidermis and an inner layer called the dermis. The surface of the skin, or the epidermis, consists of dead cells, which are rubbed off as you move, wear clothes and wash. This layer of dead cells is often referred to as 'false' skin. Just below, in the dermis, the cells are very much alive. The cells of the dermis continually multiply to replace those cells that are worn away.

Fig. 4.07 *The skin and its structures*

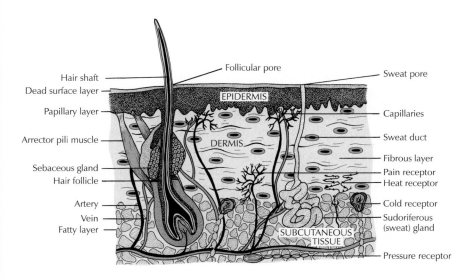

Hair shaft
Dead surface layer
Papillary layer
Arrector pili muscle
Sebaceous gland
Hair follicle
Artery
Vein
Fatty layer

Follicular pore
EPIDERMIS
DERMIS
SUBCUTANEOUS TISSUE

Sweat pore
Capillaries
Sweat duct
Fibrous layer
Pain receptor
Heat receptor
Cold receptor
Sudoriferous (sweat) gland
Pressure receptor

The skin has seven main functions

1. Secretion
2. Temperature control
3. Absorption
4. Protection – from physical abrasion, bacteria, dehydration and UV radiation
5. Excretion and elimination
6. Sensation
7. Vitamin D production

Fig. 4.08 *The epidermis*

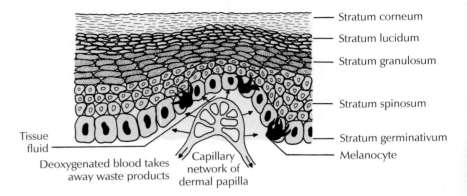

The epidermis

The epidermis consists of five layers:

1. Stratum germinativum – is the deepest layer of the epidermis. The epidermal cells originate from this layer and new cells are continually produced. Some of these cells make the protein, keratin, which toughens them. Others produce melanin, the substance that gives skin colour. As the cells in this layer increase in number, they are pushed upward and become part of the stratum granulosum.

2. Stratum spinosum – this layer is also known as the prickle cell layer, because the cells have prickle-like threads that join them together. The cells in this layer are living and contain nuclei.

3. Stratum granulosum – as the cells move up towards the surface of the skin, the cells become flattened. A substance called keratohyaline is formed which gives the skin its white appearance. The process of keratinisation begins in this area; this is the change from living, moist, nucleated cells into dead, flat, horny flakes of keratin. Keratin is also found in hair and fingernails.

4. Stratum lucidum – this layer is almost transparent in appearance. It is only a few cells thick and is believed to be the water barrier zone.

5. Stratum corneum – is the outer layer of the epidermis. It is composed of flat, dead cells, which have lost their nuclei. It is constantly being rubbed off as you move, wear clothes and wash. Keratin is also found in the cells of the stratum corneum and prevents evaporation. It also helps to ward off injury because of its toughness.

> **REMEMBER**
> The epidermis consists of five layers.

Keratinisation

There is continuous movement and change in each layer of the epidermis. Skin cells start as moist, nucleated cells and end up as dead, flat flakes, which are shed in a process called desquamation. New cells formed in the stratum germinativum migrate up through the layers to replace lost cells. This process is called keratinisation. When young it usually takes about 15 days for new cells to move upwards. This process slows down as we become older. The sun's ultraviolet rays penetrate the epidermis and effect both the new epidermal cell production and the process of keratinisation. Colour pigmentation cells in the stratum germinativum convert protein into pigment known as melanin. Melanin is the dark pigment that produces a suntan, and is a natural defence against UV rays. The cells, which form the pigment, are called melanocytes. They are spider shaped with long irregular 'arms', which reach out from the cell body. The arms of the melanocytes link with the surrounding cells. The melanocytes inject pigment granules melanosomes into cells, spreading pigment throughout the skin. Melanocytes make up about 1% of all skin cells.

> **REMEMBER**
> Melanin is the dark pigment that produces a suntan.

The dermis

The dermis, or corium, is the thick, relatively soft, innermost tissue of the skin. It shields and repairs injured tissues and is about four times thicker than the epidermis. The dermis consists mainly of the protein collagen which builds scar tissue to mend cuts and abrasions. The dermis nourishes the epidermis, and contains nerve endings and blood vessels, and may contain some fatty tissue. The bases of hairs are also located in the dermis. Underneath the dermis is a fatty subcutaneous layer. The dermis itself is divided into two layers:

The papillary layer

Has cone-like projections (papillae), which fit into corresponding depressions in the epidermis. The papillae projecting into the epidermis create contours in the skin's surface called friction ridges. It has a rich blood supply which provides the living layers of the epidermis with nutrients and allows heat to radiate to the skin's surface.

The reticular layer

A dense fibrous layer that contains proteins, fibres and the main components of the skin:

- Glands
- Hair follicles
- Muscles
- Nerve endings

A number of glands are also found in the dermis:

Sweat (sudiferous) glands

Found in the dermis, they are exocrine glands which secrete perspiration through pores onto the skin's surface. There are two types:

- Eccrine sweat glands – are found on most body surfaces but are most numerous on the scalp, palms and soles of the feet. Eccrine sweat is slightly acid, 5.73–6.49 pH and is made up of 99% water and 1% solids (sodium chloride, urea, lactic acid, amino acid, glucose and vitamins).

- Apocrine sweat glands – produce a thick milky sweat. Apocrine glands are less numerous than eccrine glands. They are concentrated in the groin, underarm, breast and genital regions and open into hair follicles. Apocrine sweat is neutral or slightly acid and consists of proteins, sugars, ammonia, ferric ions and fatty acids. Bacterial action on the constituents of apocrine sweat may produce an odour.

Sebaceous glands
Sebaceous glands are exocrine glands and secrete an oil called sebum. They are found in the dermis usually attached to the side of the hair follicle. They are found all over the body except the palms of hands and soles of feet. They are most concentrated on the scalp, chest, breasts, genital area, upper back, neck, forehead, nose and chin. Sebum is a natural lubricant that keeps the epidermis smooth and supple, and prevents it from cracking. Sebum is slightly antiseptic and waterproofs the skin. It combines with sweat to form a protective acid mantle.

Disorders
- Excessive sebum production can lead to comedones, acne and sebaceous cysts.
- Under-production of sebum can lead to flaky dry skin.

Skin cancer
There are three main types of skin cancer:

1. Basal cell carcinoma – is the least malignant and most common type of skin cancer. It is associated with long-term exposure to the sun and is therefore most likely to occur on sun-exposed areas like the head and neck.
2. Squamous cell carcinoma – squamous cells are usually found on the surface of the body, on the top layer of the skin. Squamous cell carcinoma is said to be caused by exposure to sunlight, chemicals or physical irritants. It starts off small but grows rapidly, becoming raised.
3. Malignant melanoma – this is a malignant tumour of melanocytes. It usually develops in a previously benign mole. The mole becomes larger and ulcerated and the tumour eventually spreads.

The danger signs to look out for are:

- The appearance of a new mole
- A mole that gets bigger
- A mole that bleeds, itches or ulcerates
- A mole that gets darker or lighter in colour

Hair
There are three types of hair:

1. Lanugo hair – occurs on foetuses and acts as insulation where there is a lack of body fat. It is usually shed at 36–40 weeks gestation, and is replaced by vellus hair.
2. Vellus hair – is short, soft, downy hair that is often blonde or lacks pigment. It grows in most areas of the body on both sexes.

3. Terminal hair – longer and coarser than vellus hair. It lies deep in the skin, has a strong blood supply and, unlike vellus hair, has associated sebaceous glands.

The structure of hair

Hair is composed mainly of keratin, the same protein that makes up fingernails and occurs in skin. Hair is made up of three layers:

1. The cuticle – the tough, outer protective layer of the hair. The cells are translucent and allow colour from beneath to show through. They form scales, which overlap away from the skin towards the hair tip.
2. The cortex – this is the main part of the hair that contains the colour pigment, melanin. The cells in the cortex contain bundles of fibres. The strength, thickness and elasticity of the hair is determined by the way these cells and fibres are held together. Keratin is formed in the cortex.
3. The medulla – the centre area of the hair has loosely connected, keratinised cells, interspersed with airspaces. These create the colour tones by influencing the reflection of light.

The hair grows from a narrow, tube-like depression in the skin called the hair follicle. The base of the hair follicle surrounds the hair papilla. This area has an abundant supply of blood vessels which supply nutrients and oxygen to the hair. Each papilla is surrounded by germ cells which develop into a bulb and grow to form a hair. Hairs are soft at the base but gradually harden and die as they approach the surface.

The hair growth cycle

This is the cycle of growth and replacement. The hair stops growing when it is removed from its source of nourishment, the dermal papilla. During the cycle the papilla degenerates, the blood supply ceases and the hair falls out. Eventually a new hair is formed with an active blood supply and the cycle of events leading to the growth of a new hair is repeated.

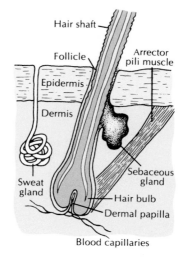

Fig. 4.09 *A hair and its follicle*

> **REMEMBER**
> Hair is made up of three layers: cuticle, cortex and medulla.

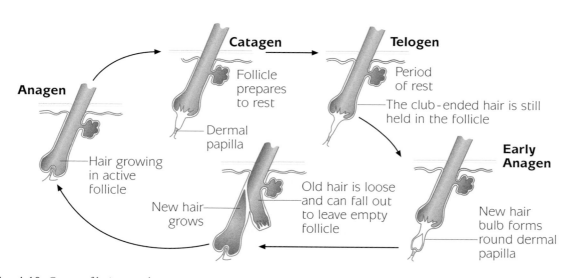

Fig. 4.10 *Stages of hair growth*

There are three stages of growth:

1. Anagen – this is the active growing stage which may last from several months to several years. The follicle comes to life and grows with nourishment from the dermal papilla.
2. Catagen – during this stage the dermal papilla detaches itself from the matrix and the follicle shrinks upwards. Slowly, the hair is detached and is shed. Its root remains in the upper follicle.
3. Telogen – this is the resting stage, when all that remains is the collection of hair germ cells from the outer root sheath, and the dermal papilla cells. It is these cells from which the new follicles will grow.

REMEMBER
The three stages of growth include anagen, catagen and telogen.

The physiological and psychological effects of massage on the integumentary system

- Nourishes the skin and its structures (through increased blood circulation)
- Improves the action of sweat and sebaceous glands (ensuring the elimination of waste)
- Improves the condition and tone of skin texture making it softer and smoother
- As dead skin cells are removed, pores are encouraged to stay open allowing increased skin respiration, suppleness and elasticity, giving the skin a healthy and glowing appearance after the treatment
- Aids desquamation (shedding of dead skin cells)
- Dilates surface capillaries and produces hyperaenmia and temporary erythema which improve the colour of the skin
- Sebaceous glands are stimulated to produce and release more sebum which lubricates the skin to keep it soft and supple
- Sweat glands are also stimulated to produce more sweat which helps in the cleansing process, and eliminates waste

REMEMBER
Massage helps to nourish the skin and all its structures.

The lymphatic system

This is a system of blind-ended vessels and lymph nodes (glands). It is considered part of the circulatory system since it consists of lymph, a moving fluid that comes from the blood, and returns to the blood by way of the lymphatic vessels. Lymph carries some nutrients around the body, especially fat. It also distributes germ-fighting white blood cells.

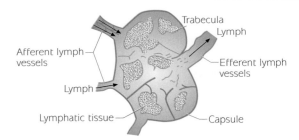

Fig. 4.11 *Lymph node section*

Lymph resembles plasma, but is more diluted and contains only about 5% of proteins and 1% of salts and extractives. It is formed from parts of blood and interstitial fluid (or tissue fluid) that collect in the spaces between cells. Some of the interstitial fluid goes back into the body through the capillary membrane, but most enters the lymphatic capillaries to become lymph. Along with this interstitial fluid, the lymph also picks up any particles that are too big to be absorbed through the capillary membrane. These include cell debris, fat globules and tiny protein particles. The lymph then moves into the larger lymphatic vessels, through the lymph nodes, and eventually enters the blood through the veins in the neck region. The lymphatic system is therefore a secondary transport system.

REMEMBER
As muscles contract they squeeze lymph through lymph vessels.

Lymph has no pump of its own. Its flow depends on pressure from the blood system and the massaging effect of the muscles. Lymph is kept moving along the lymph vessels in three ways:

1. Muscular movement, as the muscles contract they squeeze the lymph vessels and force it along.
2. Sucking action of respiration, the action of breathing.
3. Lymph vessels join together to form larger vessels and eventually form two large ducts. The right lymphatic duct collects lymph from the vessels in the head, neck and right arm. The thoracic duct collects lymph from the vessels in the left arm, lower body and chest. These two ducts join the two main veins near the heart where the lymph is reunited with the blood. Before reaching the right lymphatic duct and the thoracic duct, the lymph vessels flow into the lymph nodes/glands. The lymph always travels through the lymph nodes before entering the bloodstream; this process prevents infection and poisoning of the blood.

The spleen

The spleen is closely associated with both the circulatory and the lymphatic systems. It is an abdominal organ which lies between the stomach and the diaphragm. It plays a role in the maintenance of blood volume, production of some types of blood cells, and recovery of material from worn-out red blood cells. It is also involved in the removal of blood cells and bacteria from the blood. The spleen forms red blood cells in the foetus and works with the bone marrow to produce extra red cells after blood loss due to severe injury or impairment of the bone marrow. It separates worn-out blood cells from the blood stream and manufactures lymphocytes.

The physiological and psychological effects of massage on the lymphatic and immune system

- Stimulates the lymphatic flow
- Improved elimination of impurities from the body
- Helps in the removal of lactic acid and other waste
- Increases white blood cell production which helps to strengthen the immune system
- When we sustain injuries there is often oedema (swelling) which should be dispersed into the lymphatic circulation. Massage can help empty the lymph vessels and allow the swelling to disperse

The squeezing, compressive and pushing components of massage bring about the drainage of lymph in the same way that it assists the movement of blood in the superficial veins. Massage movements compress the soft walls of the lymphatic vessels and the lymph within them is pushed onwards. Pressure from massage increases the interstitial pressure and aids absorption of tissue fluid across the capillary walls. The tissue fluid contains nutrients and oxygen that feed the tissues, thus the appearance of the area being massaged is improved. If the lymphatic circulation becomes stagnant the waste products accumulate, the area they collect in can become swollen and puffy, and the skin can appear uneven in texture, dull and blemished. Therefore a massage can help relieve these conditions.

Petrissage movements squeeze the lymph from the spaces and the effleurage moves it on to the nearest lymph glands. The therapist must remember that the lymph nodes which produce lymphatic fluid are located underneath all the joints of the body, and by rubbing and applying circular movement one can stimulate these lymph nodes.

The ancient Indians felt that the benefits of massage were medicated by increasing the flow of lymph in lymph vessels and ascribed to lymph the properties of increased viscosity, nourishment, solidarity and sexual stamina.

The muscular system

The human body contains more than 650 individual muscles anchored to the skeleton, which provide pulling power so that you can move around. These muscles constitute about 40% of your total body weight. Each muscle's points of attachment to bones or other muscles is known as the point of origin or insertion.

The point of origin is the point where the muscle is anchored to a bone. The point of insertion is the point where the muscle attaches to the bone it moves. Generally, the muscles are attached by tough fibrous structures called tendons. These attachments bridge one or more joints, and the result of muscle contraction is the movement of these joints.

Primarily, muscle groups move the body, not individual muscles. Groups of muscles power actions ranging from the threading of a needle to the lifting of heavy weights.

Structure

Muscle tissue is bound together in bundles and contained in a sheath. The end of the sheath extends to form a tendon that attaches muscle to the other parts of the body. Muscle is 75% water, 20% proteins and 5% fats, mineral salts and glycogen.

Function

The function of muscle is to produce movement, maintain posture and provide heat for the body.

There are three types of muscular tissue, each of which has a different function and structure:

1. Involuntary muscle (also known as smooth muscle)
    These are the muscles we do not consciously control, for example, those found in the walls of blood and lymphatic vessels, and in respiratory, digestive and genito-urinary systems. The cells of the muscles are spindle-shaped, with no distinct membrane and only one nucleus.
2. Voluntary muscle (also known as skeletal or striated muscle)
    These are muscles which we consciously control, for example those in our arms and legs. They consist of bundles of muscle fibres, striped in appearance and enclosed in a sheath (fascia). Voluntary muscle has cylindrical cells which make up the fibres. Each fibre has several nuclei. The stripes are made of proteins (actin and myosin filaments) which run across the muscle fibres in transverse bands. They are alternately light and dark and give voluntary muscle its other name: striated. When the muscle contracts the actin filaments slide between the myosin filaments and cause a shortening and thickening of the fibres.

3. Cardiac muscle
   This is a specialised tissue found only in the heart. Its function is to power the pump action of the heart. It is involuntary muscle tissue but its fibres are striated and each cell has one nucleus.

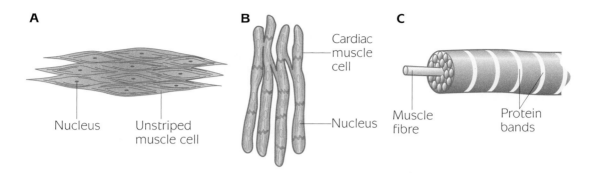

Fig. 4.12 *Three types of muscle in the body*

Blood supply
Blood vessels bring glucose and oxygen to supply energy and the calcium ions necessary for normal contraction. They remove waste products like lactic acid and carbon dioxide. Blood also brings adrenaline which aids muscle contraction.

Nerve supply
All muscle tissue must be well supplied with nerves for contraction. In skeletal muscle, nerves bring the impulses which stimulate the muscle tissue to contract according to the all-or-nothing principle. This is where either all or no muscle fibres contract.

Muscle fibres
They are long, thin, multi-nucleated cells. The fibres vary from 10 to 100 microns in diameter, and from a few millimetres to a number of centimetres in length. The long fibres extend the full length of the muscle while the short fibres end in connective tissue intersections within the muscle.

Muscle attachments
A muscle has two or more points of attachment known as the origin and insertion of the muscle. The origin is usually proximal and stationary or immoveable. The insertion is usually distal and moveable.

Muscle tone
In the living body there will be a level of partial contraction that is constantly maintained by each muscle to maintain posture and remain in a ready and active state. This muscle tone is controlled on an autonomic level through a reflex connection between the motor and sensory nerves.

Muscle fatigue
When a muscle is continuously stimulated, its contraction becomes progressively weaker and eventually can cease. This condition is called muscle fatigue and is due to the accumulation of the toxic waste products lactic acid and carbon dioxide, as well as the shortage of ATP (adenosine triphosphate, an energy-rich compound), glucose and oxygen, which provide energy for contraction.

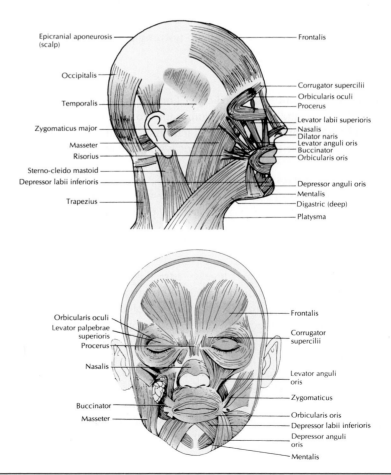

REMEMBER

A build-up of lactic acid can cause fibrositis.

When skeletal muscles are very fatigued, the muscles exert very little balancing effect. Therefore the tendons and ligaments will have to support the body and as a result may become strained. A build-up of lactic acid can also cause a condition called fibrositis, where there is stiffness, pain and inflammation in the affected muscle.

Muscles of the face and neck

- The sterno-cleido mastoid muscle is located in the neck. It is a thin, broad muscle that narrows at the centre. It originates from two heads, one from the sternum and one from the clavicle and runs upward, inserting into the mastoid (the temporal bone behind the ear). This muscle is used to tilt the head from side to side.

REMEMBER

The trapezius is a postural muscle as well as an active mover.

- The trapezius is one of the largest shoulder muscles and is the most superficial muscle on the back of the neck and upper trunk. It is a broad, flat, triangular muscle that lies just below the skin and covers the upper back part of the neck and shoulders. It links the neck with the spine (dorsal vertebrae), ribs and shoulder bones (scapula). This muscle is used to turn and tilt the head, raise and twist the arms, and to shrug or steady the shoulders.

There are about thirty muscles associated with facial expression, controlling the eyes, face and mouth. These muscles take their origin from the bones of the facial skeleton and attach to the soft tissues of the facial skin, such as the eyelids, nose, cheeks and lips. Some muscles open these orifices wide, others narrow or close them. There are seventeen

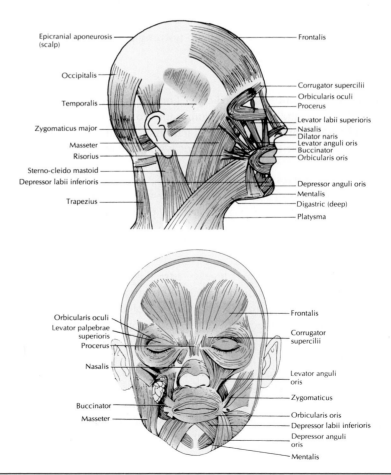

Fig. 4.13 *Muscles of the face and neck*

muscles used for smiling. Branches of two main nerves, the right and left facial nerves, which arise from the brain stem, supply all the muscles of the face. These branches of the facial nerve control the muscle movements of the face.

- The occipito-frontalis is a broad muscular-fibrous layer that covers the epicranium (top of the skull). It consists of two thin layers of muscle. The occipital portion, sometimes called the occipitalis muscle, is quadrilateral in form and about an inch and a half in length. It covers the back of the cranium (skull). The frontal portion, sometimes called the frontalis, is also quadrilateral in form. It is broader and its fibres are longer and it covers the forehead. The frontalis and occipitalis portions of the muscle are joined together by a thin, flat intermediate tendon called the galia aponeurotica. The aponeurosis is located above the occipito and frontalis muscles and covers the top of the cranium. It works with the occipito-frontalis muscles to move the scalp. The frontalis muscle elevates the eyebrows and draws the scalp forward.

- The orbicularis oculi muscle is also known as the orbicularis palpebrarum muscle. It is a sphincter muscle, or ring-shaped muscle, that covers the eyelid and surrounds the orbit of each eye. The muscle is composed of two parts, one of which covers the eyelid, the other surrounds the orbit. The two portions work together to narrow the eye, thus causing the eye to close or blink.

- The zygomaticus minor is a slender cheek muscle. It arises from the malar bone and extends downward and inward, and is inserted into the angle of the mouth. It lies just in front of the zygomaticus major muscle and draws the upper lip backward, upward and outward and is used in expressing sadness.

- The zygomaticus major is another slender cheek muscle. It arises from the malar bone and extends downward and inward, and is inserted into the angle of the mouth. It draws the upper lip upward and outward and is used in smiling.

- The risorius muscle is a narrow bundle of fibres. It originates from the fascia just above the masseter muscle, and extends horizontally forward to insert in the skin at the angle of the mouth. This muscle retracts the angles of the mouth.

- The platysma muscle is a broad, thin sheet of muscle that originates in the pectoral and deltoid (chest and shoulder) muscles. It runs upward over the collarbone and inward along each side of the neck. This muscle works to draw the lower lips and corner of the mouth sideways and down, partially opening the mouth. It is used when expressing surprise, fear or horror. It also increases the diameter of the neck as seen during intense breathing from fast running.

- The mentalis muscle arises from the front of the lower jaw below the roots of the teeth, extends upward covering the chin, and inserts into the lower lip. It lies just underneath the depressor labii inferioris. The muscle raises the fleshy part of the chin, which in turn pushes up the lower lip as when expressing sadness, anger or doubt.

- The orbicularis oris lies between the skin and the mucous membrane of the lips. It has no bone attachment. Muscle fibres surround the mouth and extend upwards to the septum of the nose and downwards to the region between the lower lip and chin. These muscular fibres are partially derived from other facial muscles that are inserted into the lips. The orbicularis oris pulls the lips against the teeth and causes lips to close and pucker, as when kissing.

- The buccinator is a broad thin muscle with a quadrilateral form and is supplied by the facial nerve. This cheek muscle is located on each side of the face in the space between the jaws. The muscle compresses the cheeks and works with the tongue to keep food between the teeth when chewing.
- The masseter muscle is located on the side of the jaw. It extends from the zygomatic bone to the ramus of the mandible (jaw). It is one of the chewing muscles that elevate the mandible, and pull the mouth shut. It is also used when we talk. The mandibular branch of the trigeminal nerve innervates the masseter.
- The temporalis muscle is a flat, fan-shaped muscle located in the temple. It arises in the temporal fossa and fills the depression on the side of the skull. It inserts on the coronoid process of the mandible and the front edge of the ramus of the mandible. This muscle pulls the jaw upward which closes the jaw and helps to clench your teeth for chewing.

Muscles that move the shoulder and arms

- The deltoid is a large, thick, powerful muscle. It is triangular in form with a coarse texture. On its broad side, it originates from the clavicle (collar bone) and from the scapula (shoulder blade) and inserts in the humerus (upper arm bone). It covers the outer side of the shoulder joint, giving the shoulder its rounded appearance. This muscle moves the humerus bone and is used to raise the arm outward from the side. It works with the pectoralis major to move the arm forward, and with the teres major and latissimus dorsi to move the arm back.
- The pectoralis major muscle is located at the front of the thoracic cage. It is a thick, fan-shaped muscle and is divided into two parts that begin at the armpit and cover most of the front of the chest. The upper, or clavicular, part is attached to the clavicle. The lower, or sternocostal portion, is attached mainly to the sternum (and costal cartilage). This muscle is used when you bring your arms across the chest, raise and lower the arms and rotate the arms. The clavicular portion will raise the arm, while the sternocostal portion will pull it down.

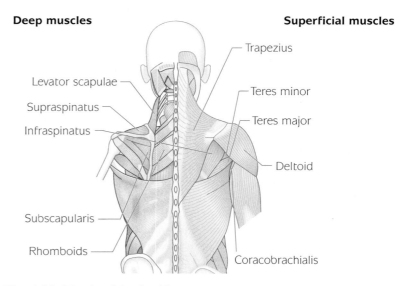

Deep muscles   **Superficial muscles**

Trapezius

Levator scapulae

Supraspinatus

Infraspinatus

Teres minor

Teres major

Deltoid

Subscapularis

Rhomboids

Coracobrachialis

Fig. 4.14 *Muscles of the shoulders*

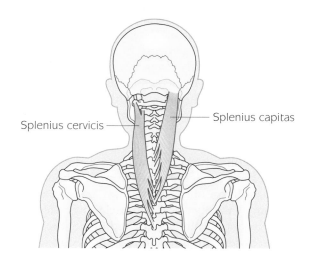

Fig. 4.14 *Muscles of the shoulders (cont)*

Splenius cervicis

Splenius capitas

- The serratus anterior (serratus magnus) is a large quadrilateral muscle that curves along the rib cage. The muscle is divided into several bundles, each of which extends along the side and upper border of each rib. The muscle is divided into two portions, an upper and lower portion. The upper portion lies along the upper side of the rib cage and the armpit. The lower portion consists of five or six pointed digitations, which create a fan-shaped mass extending from the scapula. This muscle is used every time you reach out or push forward with your arms. It also helps raise the shoulder joint when lifting your arm above your head.

- The latissimus dorsi is a wide, flat muscle located on the lower half of the back. The muscle fibres at its tip insert under the scapula (shoulder blade) and join to the humerus (upper arm bone) in the shoulder. The base of this triangular muscle is attached along the lumbar and lower half of the thoracic vertebrae (spine), the lower ribs, and even the hipbones far below. This muscle gives your arms motion. It is used when swimming or when you swing your arms back when jogging. It is also used to reach up to grab something above your head.

- The levator scapula lies along the back and side part of the neck. It originates deep in the side of the neck near the base of the skull, passes down and inserts in the scapula. As the name implies, this muscle is the 'shoulder blade lifter'. This muscle tenses up, becoming hard and stiff, when you carry a weight on your shoulder.

- The rhomboids major and the rhomboids minor form a flat, quadrilateral muscle in the upper back that lie under the trapezius. The muscles extend from the spine to the edge of the scapula. They are barely separable as two muscles. These muscles assist in rotating the scapula and supporting the head. When you sneeze, the shoulder, back and abdominal muscles contract quickly to force air out of the nasal passages, while the rhombodeus major and minor muscles hold your head and neck steady.

- The triceps brachii (three-headed muscle) lies at the upper portion of the inside of the arm. It is the main extensor of the arm and is made up of three teardrop-shaped heads: the long head, the lateral head and the medial head. When working with other nearby muscles it can also move the shoulder, as its upper ends are attached to the scapula. The long head, the largest of the three heads, is attached to the scapula just below the rounded socket of the shoulder joint, and extends almost three-quarters of the way towards the front of the arm. The lateral head lies on the back and side of the upper arm. The medial head curves around the back of the humerus and is mostly covered by the long head. The lower end is attached to the flattened end of the ulna. The triceps brachii extends the forearm at the elbow joint. It works with the biceps brachii to control the up and down movement of the forearm.

Arm muscles

- The biceps brachii (two-headed arm muscle) consists of the long head and the short head. It extends from the shoulder to the elbow and is the main flexor of the elbow joint. Like the triceps brachii, when working with other nearby muscles, it can also move the shoulder, as its upper ends are attached to the scapula. In addition it can twist the lower arm so that the palm faces outward, a movement called supination. At the lower end, the biceps tapers into a flat, strong tendon that is firmly fixed to a bulge on the upper end of the radius. The biceps and the triceps work together to control the up and down movement of the forearm.

The muscles of the trunk

Fig. 4.15 *Muscles of the anterior trunk*

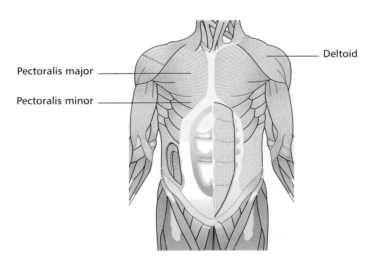

Fig. 4.16 *Muscles of the back*

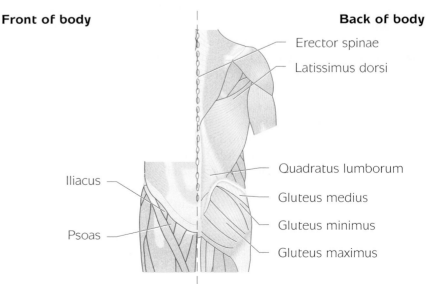

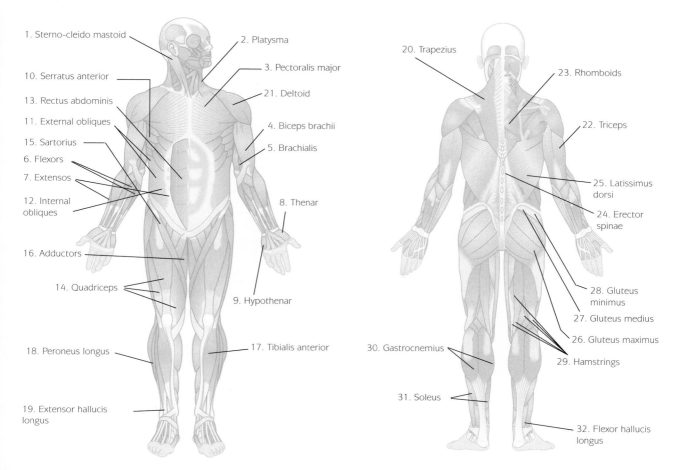

Fig. 4.17 *Anterior view*

1. Sterno-cleido mastoid
10. Serratus anterior
13. Rectus abdominis
11. External obliques
15. Sartorius
6. Flexors
7. Extensos
12. Internal obliques
16. Adductors
14. Quadriceps
18. Peroneus longus
19. Extensor hallucis longus
2. Platysma
3. Pectoralis major
21. Deltoid
4. Biceps brachii
5. Brachialis
8. Thenar
9. Hypothenar
17. Tibialis anterior

Fig. 4.18 *Posterior view*

20. Trapezius
23. Rhomboids
22. Triceps
25. Latissimus dorsi
24. Erector spinae
28. Gluteus minimus
27. Gluteus medius
26. Gluteus maximus
29. Hamstrings
30. Gastrocnemius
31. Soleus
32. Flexor hallucis longus

The physiological and psychological effects of massage on the muscular system

- Muscles are nourished, strengthened and toned
- Helps to increase muscles' metabolism and remove lactic acid and other waste
- Helps to relieve muscle fatigue, reduce pain and stiffness
- Aids tissue repair and recovery
- Muscles maintain a balance in relaxing. Some massage movements relax and stretch the muscles and soft tissues of the body, reducing muscular tension and cramp. Weak neck muscles are the chief reason for forward head posture, which could lead to rounded shoulders and stooping.
- Aids in the breakdown of adhesions and fibrostic nodules that may have developed as a result of tension, poor posture or injury

Fig. 4.19 *Overview of the nervous system*

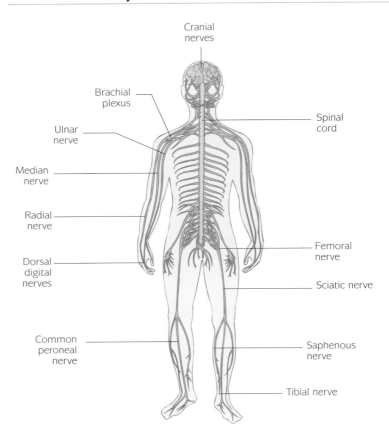

The neurological or nervous system transmits and receives messages to and from the brain and all parts of the body. It works with the endocrine system to maintain homeostasis.

The main parts are:

- The central nervous system – also known as the cerebrospinal system because it consists of the brain and the spinal cord
- The peripheral nervous system – consisting of 12 pairs of cranial nerves arising from the brain, and 31 pairs of spinal nerves arising from the spinal cord
- The autonomic nervous system – supplies nerves to all the body's internal organs. The autonomic nervous system is split into the sympathetic and parasympathetic nervous system.

REMEMBER
The central nervous system consists of the brain and spinal cord.

The central nervous system
The brain
The brain is at the centre of the central nervous system and fills the cranium. It is the main mass exercising control over the body and mind. The brain is well protected from the outside by the hard bone structure of the skull. Inside, the brain is protected by three membranes called the meninges:

- The dura mater (strong or hard mother) – the outer layer which is constructed of strong fibrous tissue anchored to the skull.

- The arachnoid mater – the middle layer which is more delicate than the dura mater and is not anchored to the skull. Beneath it is a large reservoir of cerebral spinal fluid which surrounds the brain and on which it rests.
- The pia mater – the inner layer which is a thin vascular membrane that is in contact with grey matter of the brain itself, and dips deep down between the brain convolutions.

The adult human brain weighs around 1360g and is so full of water that it tends to slump rather like a blancmange if placed without the support of a firm surface. It is estimated that it has 12 billion nerve cells or neurons.

The spinal cord
The spinal cord is the other main part of the central nervous system. It consists of white matter on the surface and grey matter inside. The spinal cord carries motor and sensory nerve fibres along its length, sending messages about feeling and movement to and from the body and brain.

The peripheral nervous system
The peripheral nervous system constitutes the nervous system outside the central nervous system. It contains motor and sensory nerves which transmit information to and from the body and brain. It consists of 12 pairs of cranial nerves, 31 pairs of spinal nerves and the autonomic nervous system.

The autonomic nervous system
This controls all body structures over which we have no voluntary control. It is divided into two separate parts:

1. The sympathetic system – comprises a gangliated cord, which runs on either side of the front of the vertebral column. The principal plexuses of this system are:

   - The cardiac plexus which supplies all the thoracic viscera and the thoracic vessels
   - The solar plexus which supplies all the abdominal viscera
   - The hypogastric plexus, which supplies the pelvic organs.

   It stimulates the action of organs, releases noradrenaline to prepare the body for excitement and stress (fight or flight sysndrome), accelerates the heart rate, causes dilation of the arteries and other blood vessels, raises blood pressure, and restricts blood flow to the digestive system.

2. The parasympathetic nervous system consists mainly of the vagus nerve which gives off branches to the organs of the thorax and abdomen. It also includes branches from other cranial nerves, mainly the third, seventh and ninth, as well as nerves in the sacral region of the spinal column. It slows down the action of organs, releases a neurotransmitter, and slows the action of the heart as well as constricting blood flow to the heart muscles.

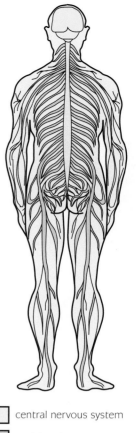

central nervous system

peripheral nervous system

Fig. 4.20 *The central nervous system*

The physiological and psychological effects of massage on the nervous system

- A slow and rhythmical massage helps to relax the nerves
- A faster massage helps to increase mental alertness
- The effects may be soothing and sedative providing relief from nervous irritability (invaluable in cases of insomnia and tension headaches)
- Helps to stimulate nerves, promoting an increase in the activity of muscles, vessels and glands governed by them (invaluable in cases of lethargy and fatigue)
- Creates a feeling of wellbeing and health
- Promotes feelings of vigour and increases energy
- Increases postural awareness
- Promotes feelings of being cared for which promotes relaxation and a sense of wellbeing
- Reduces mental stress which enhances feelings of contentment and relaxation

The reproductive system

The reproductive system is the process by which new individuals of a species are produced and genetic material is passed from generation to generation. This ensures continuation of the species.

Fig. 4.21 *The reproductive organs of a man*

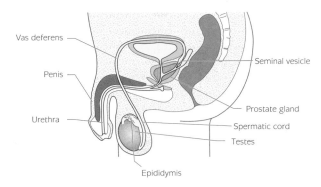

The organs of the male reproductive system are the testes, a system of ducts, accessory sex glands, and several supporting structures, including the penis. The male reproductive system depends on both hormonal and neural mechanisms to function correctly.

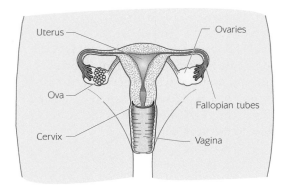

Fig. 4.22 *The reproductive organs of a woman*

The female reproduction organs include the ovaries, vagina, uterus, external genital organs and mammary glands, and others. As in the male, female reproduction is under the control of hormonal and nervous regulation.

There are reproductive hormones in males and females (e.g. testosterone, oestrogens, progesterone which have a source (e.g. part of the testes, ovaries, hypothalamus) and target tissue (like the testes and uterus) in order to get a response (e.g. stimulation of testosterone, development of mammary glands). Endocrine and nervous systems are at the helm of the reproductive system

The physiological and psychological effects of massage on the reproductive system

The use of abdominal and back massage can help to alleviate menstrual problems such as period pains, irregular menstruation, PMS and symptoms of menopause.

The respiratory system

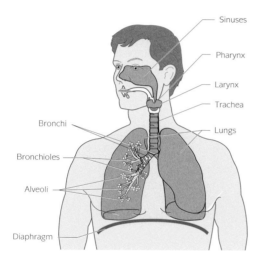

Fig. 4.23 *Respiratory organs*

The respiratory system consists of the nasal cavity, pharynx, larynx, trachea, bronchi and lungs. Respiratory movements are accomplished by the diaphragm and the muscles of the thoracic wall. Oxygen is essential for all the cells of the body and carbon dioxide is a major waste product. Both the cardiovascular and respiratory systems take oxygen from the air and transport it to individual cells. They also transport carbon dioxide from cells and release it from the body back into the air.

REMEMBER
Oxygen is essential for all the cells.

Respiration involves several important processes:

1. Ventilation – the movement of air into and out of respiratory passages and the lungs
2. Gas exchange – between the air in the lungs and the blood
3. Transport – of oxygen and carbon dioxide in the blood
4. Gas – exchange between the blood and the tissues

The muscles of inspiration and of expiration have their own actions. Muscles of inspiration elevate the ribs and thorax, and compress the abdomen.

Oxygen is transported from the lungs to the tissues in a chemical combination with haemoglobin in the red blood cells. Respiration is controlled by neurones in nervous system mechanisms.

The physiological and psychological effects of massage on the respiratory system

- Increases blood flow to lungs (producing a better interchange of gases)
- Helps loosen mucus and eases congestion
- Increases lung activity making them more resistant to infections
- Massage helps to slow and deepen the breath therefore helping the body to relax

The skeletal system

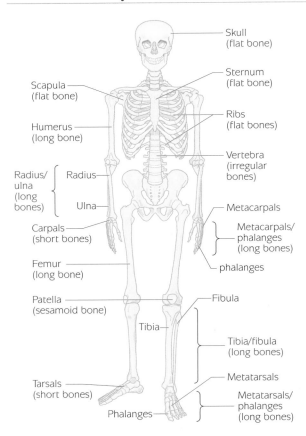

Skull (flat bone)
Sternum (flat bone)
Scapula (flat bone)
Ribs (flat bones)
Humerus (long bone)
Vertebra (irregular bones)
Radius/ulna (long bones)
Radius
Ulna
Metacarpals
Metacarpals/phalanges (long bones)
Carpals (short bones)
phalanges
Femur (long bone)
Patella (sesamoid bone)
Fibula
Tibia
Tibia/fibula (long bones)
Tarsals (short bones)
Metatarsals
Metatarsals/phalanges (long bones)
Phalanges

Fig. 4.24 *The skeletal system*

The skeleton is the framework of the human anatomy. It supports the body and protects its internal organs. The skeletal system is made of connective tissue, bone and cartilage and consists of a large number of separate structures (the bones) which articulate (meet at a joint) with one another. The skeleton is made up of 206 bones, about half of which are in the hands and feet. Most of the bones are connected to other bones at flexible joints, which lend the framework a high degree of flexibility. Only one bone, the hyoid, is not directly connected to another bone. It anchors the tongue and is attached to the styloid processes of the skull by a ligament. The skeletons of male and female bodies are essentially the same. The only noteworthy exceptions are that female bones are usually lighter and thinner than male bones, and the female pelvis is shallower and wider than the male. This latter difference serves to make childbirth easier.

The spinal column

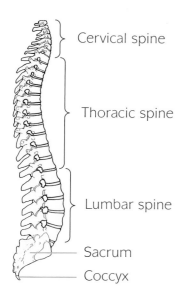

Cervical spine

Thoracic spine

Lumbar spine

Sacrum

Coccyx

Fig. 4.25 *Bones of the vertebral column*

The spinal, or vertebral column, is one of the primary support structures for the human skeleton. It consists of 24 bones split into three sections: seven cervical vertebrae form the neck, 12 thoracic vertebrae form the upper back, and five lumbar vertebrae form the lower back. The vertebrae are irregularly shaped and stack together. They are separated by intervertebral discs, consisting of an outer rim of fibrocartilage and a central core of soft, gelatinous material. They act as shock absorbers and the cartilaginous joints they form contribute to the flexibility of the vertebral column as a whole. Beneath the vertebrae is the sacrum (five fixed bones) and the coccyx (four fused bones). Made up of separate, pseudo-separate, and fused vertebrae, the spine features a great deal of articulation. This allows support and movement of the skull, flexion of the neck and back, provides anchor sites for the ribs (which enclose the abdominal cavity), and supports and protects the spinal cord. Tough bands of fibrous tissue and ligaments hold the vertebrae together and help maintain the intervertebral discs in position. They also control the degree of flexibility in the spine.

The typical vertebrae has a body of solid bony material, which supports the weight of the spine, and an arch which forms the vertebral foramen. It is the adjoining vertebral foramina which create a canal running through the spinal column which houses and protects the spinal cord, the primary nerve pathway to and from the brain.

The transverse processes
Most vertebrae exhibit pronounced lateral protrusions (or processes), one on each side of the vertebra. These transverse processes serve as the attachment sites for ligaments (intertransverse ligaments) and muscles, which control the bending and twisting of the vertebral column. The base of each transverse process, in most vertebrae, is just off the main body of the vertebra, located at the pedicle. The pedicle is part of the ring-like

> **REMEMBER**
> The spine is made up of three sections, the cervical, thoracic and lumbar.

structure of a vertebra, which also includes the body and lamina of a vertebra, forming the vertebral foramen.

Cervical vertebrae

The cervical vertebrae are the first (upper) seven in the vertebral column. The first cervical vertebra is the atlas, the second is called the axis. The other five cervical vertebrae have no names, but are called by their number (e.g. third cervical vertebra). Each of the cervical vertebra features a body (anterior, or frontal, portion) and an arch (posterior, or rear, portion). The body of each vertebra in the column bears the weight of the vertebrae above it (and the skull), while the arch serves to create a canal-like area along the spine to house and protect the spinal cord. Every cervical vertebra has a foramen (opening) in each of its transverse processes. The arch of the vertebra features a small knob or prominence, called an anterior tubercle. The anterior tubercles on the sixth cervical vertebra are particularly large and are known as the carotid tubercles.

The atlas

The atlas is the first of the seven cervical vertebrae and is so called because it bears the direct weight of the skull, just as the mythical Greek hero Atlas bore the world on his shoulders. The atlas vertebra meets with the occipital condyles, which flank the foramen magnum in the basal part of the occipital bone of the skull. This junction forms the atlanto-occipital joint, and is responsible for the primary articulation between the spine and the skull. It is the only vertebra in the spine which has no vertebral body. The atlas vertebra in turn rests upon the axis vertebra, which is the second of the cervical vertebrae in the spine. The articulation between these two vertebrae occurs at lateral articular surfaces with a unique juncture between a concave facet and an upward-protruding structure on the axis, called a dens.

The axis

The axis is the second of the seven cervical vertebrae, and is called such because it allows axial (rotational) movement of the skull. The axis lies directly beneath the atlas vertebra. The articulation between the two is regulated by the alar ligament which attaches to both the atlas and axis.

The thoracic vertebrae

The thoracic vertebrae are the middle twelve in the vertebral column. Most of the thoracic vertebrae feature costal facets on the body, that is, surfaces that articulate with the ribs. The thoracic vertebrae have no foramina in the transverse processes (as the cervical vertebrae have), a spinous process which points back and down, and a round vertebral foramen. Some rotation can occur between the thoracic vertebrae, but their connection with the ribs prevents much movement.

The lumbar vertebrae

The lumbar vertebrae are the five vertebrae which are below the thoracic vertebrae and above the fused vertebrae of the sacrum. The lumbar vertebrae feature no facets on the body or transverse processes (as the thoracic vertebrae have), and the bodies of the lumbar vertebrae are much larger than those of the cervical or thoracic vertebrae. The transverse processes of the lumbar vertebrae (which also represent their rib elements) lack the foramina, which characterise the cervical vertebrae.

REMEMBER
The spine is held together by ligaments.

The skeleton

The skeleton is a hard framework that supports and protects the muscles and organs of the body, and enables movement. It maintains body shape and suspends some of the internal organs. Bones act as levers and when muscle pulls on bones, parts of the body move. The result of the co-ordinated action of muscle on bone is called locomotion. Muscles are usually attached to bones by tendons, made of tough, fibrous, non-elastic connective tissue. Bones form red blood cells in the bone marrow as well as provide a reservoir of minerals, especially calcium phosphate.

Bones are living tissues made from bone-forming cells called osteoblasts. The tissue varies in density. Many bones have a central cavity containing bone marrow. This tissue is a source of most cells of the blood and also acts as storage site for fat.

The skeleton is formed of 206 bones and is divided into two parts:

1. The axial skeleton – supports the head, neck and trunk. It includes the skull, vertebral column, ribs and sternum.
2. The appendicular skeleton – supports the appendages or limbs and attaches them to the rest of the body. It includes the shoulder girdle, upper limbs, pelvic girdle and lower limbs.

The axial skeleton

Skull

The skull consists of the cranium and face. The eight most important bones of the cranium are:

◆ One frontal bone – comprises the bones of the forehead and forms the prominent ridges of the eyes.

◆ Two parietal bones – these bones form the sides and the top of the skull. The joint between them is called the sagittal suture.

◆ Two temporal bones – these lie on each side of the head and are divided into four parts: squamus part, petrous portion, mastoid process and zygomatic process.

◆ One occipital bone – forms the back of the head and the upper part of the back of the skull.

◆ One sphenoid bone – lies across the base of the skull and is rested on by the brain and the pituitary gland.

◆ One ethmoid bone – forms part of the eye cavity.

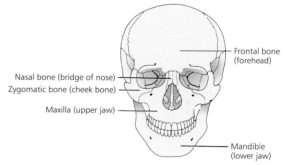

Fig. 4.26 *Bones of the skull*

The face

There are 14 bones in the face. The most important bones are:

◆ Mandible – forms the lower part of the jaw, articulates with the rest of the skull by two hinge joints, allows speech and aids chewing.

◆ Maxillae – forms the upper jaw and houses the upper teeth. Originates as two bones but are fused together before birth.

◆ Zygomatic – forms the prominence of the cheeks, part of the walls and floor of the orbital cavities.

The other bones of the face are the nasal, lacrimal, palatine, turbinate and the vomer bones.

Sinuses

Sinuses containing air are present in the sphenoid, ethmoid, maxillary and frontal bones. They communicate with the nasal cavity, and their functions are to give resonance to the voice and to lighten the bones of the face and cranium, thus making it easier for the head to balance on top of the vertebral column.

The thoracic cage

Fig. 4.27 *Bones of the upper body*

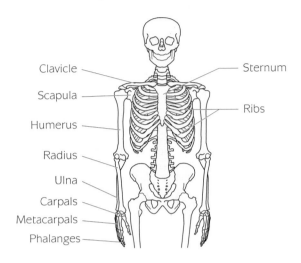

The thoracic cage consists of:

◆ One sternum – also known as the breastbone, this is a flat bone felt just under the skin in the middle and front of the chest. The manubrium is the uppermost section and articulates at the sternoclavicular joints and with the first two pairs of ribs.

◆ Twelve pairs of ribs – which form the bony lateral part of the thoracic cage and articulate posteriorly with the thoracic vertebrae. The first ten pairs are attached anteriorly to the sternum by the costal cartilages. The last two pairs of ribs are known as floating ribs as they have no anterior attachment.

◆ Twelve thoracic vertebrae – that articulate with the ribs.

Other bones that form the axial skeleton are the vertebral column, the cervical, thoracic and lumbar vertebrae, the sacrum and the coccyx. See pages 79–80 for more information.

The appendicular skeleton

The appendicular skeleton consists of the shoulder girdle with the upper limbs, and the pelvic girdle with the lower limbs.

The shoulder girdle and upper limb
Each shoulder girdle consists of:

◆ One clavicle – commonly known as the collarbone, this is a long bone with a double curve. It articulates with the manubrium of the sternum at the sternoclavicular joint and forms the acromioclavicular joint with the acromion process of the scapula. It provides the only link between the upper limb and the axial skeleton.

- One scapula – commonly known as the shoulder blade. This is a flat, triangular-shaped bone, lying on the posterior chest wall superficial to the ribs, and separated from them by muscles. At the lateral angle there is a shallow articular surface, the glenoid activity, which forms the shoulder joint together with the head of the humerus. On the posterior surface there is a spinous process that projects beyond the lateral angle of the bone that overhangs the shoulder joint, called the acromion process. It articulates with the clavicle at the acromioclavicular joint. The coracoid process, a projection from the upper border of the bone, gives attachment to muscles that move the shoulder joint.

Each upper limb consists of:

- One humerus – the bone of the upper arm. The head articulates with the glenoid cavity of the scapula, forming the shoulder joint.
- One ulna and one radius – these bones form the forearm. The ulna is longer than, and medial to, the radius. They articulate with the humerus at the elbow joint, the carpal bones at the wrist joint and with each other at the proximal and distal radioulnar joints.
- Eight carpal bones – there are eight wrist bones arranged in two rows of four.
  Proximal row – scaphoid, lunate, triquetral, pisiform. Distal row – trapezium, trapezoid, capitate, hamate.
- Five metacarpal bones – there are five bones that form the palm of the hand. They are simply numbered from the thumb side inwards.
- Fourteen phalanges – there are 14 finger bones, three in each finger and two in the thumb.

Pelvic girdle and lower limb

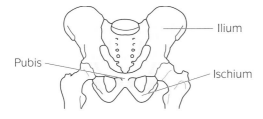

Fig. 4.28 *The pelvic girdle*

The bones of the pelvic girdle consist of:

- Two innominate bones – commonly known as hip bones, each consists of three fused bones, the ilium, ischium and pubis.
- One sacrum – the pelvis is formed by the two innominate bones which articulate anteriorly at the symphysis pubis and posteriorly with the sacrum at the sacroliliac joints.

The bones of the lower limb consist of:

- One femur – the femur is the longest and strongest bone in the whole body. The head of the femur is almost spherical and fits into the acetabulum of the hip to form the hip joint.
- One tibia – commonly known as the shin bone, the tibia is the medial of the two lower leg bones.
- One fibula – this is a long and slender bone, lateral to the leg.

> **REMEMBER**
> The pelvis of the female is wider and shallower than that of the male.

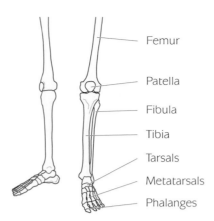

Fig. 4.29 *Bones of the lower limbs*

- One patella – the knee cap is a triangular-shaped sesamoid bone associated with the knee joint.
- Seven tarsal bones – there are seven anklebones, which form the posterior part of the foot. They consist of: one talus, one calcaneus, one navicular, three cuneiform, one cuboid.
- Five metatarsal bones – there are five bones numbered from the inside, outwards, which form the greater dorsum part of the foot.
- Fourteen phalanges of the foot – there are 14 phalanges in each foot, two in each big toe and three in each of the other toes.

Joints

Fig. 4.30 *Structure of a synovial joint*

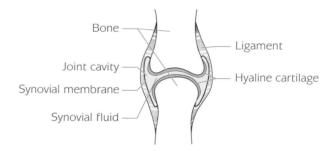

Joints are the body's hinges of which there are three types:

1. Fixed or fibrous joints, e.g. sutures in the skull, pelvic girdle
2. Slightly moveable or cartilaginous joints, e.g. spine
3. Freely moveable or synovial joints of which there are five types: ball and socket (e.g. hip joint), hinge (e.g. elbow), gliding (e.g. between tarsals and carpals), pivot (e.g. atlas and axis), saddle (only found between the phalanges of the thumb and its metacarpal).

REMEMBER
The three types of joints are known as fibrous, cartilaginous and synovial.

Postural deformities

The spine has two natural curves, an inward curve in the lower back and a slightly outward curve in the upper back. In some cases, the spine's natural curves become exaggerated, causing unnatural curves or postural deformities. They may be caused by accidents, environmental factors or by congenital defects.

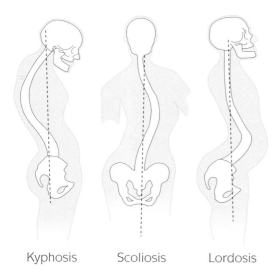

Fig. 4.31 *Postural faults*

Kyphosis   Scoliosis   Lordosis

There are three types of postural deformities:

1. Kyphosis – an exaggerated outward curvature of the spine
2. Scoliosis – a sideways curvature of the spine
3. Lordosis – an exaggerated inward curvature of the spine

Fracture
A fracture is a breakage of a bone because of injury or disease. There are a number of different types of fractures.

The physiological and psychological effects of massage on the skeletal system
- Bones are strengthened and nourished. Deep massage movements will stimulate blood flow to the periosteum (connective tissue covering the bone) therefore increasing blood supply to the bone
- Cellular regeneration is encouraged
- Disperses fluid and lubricates and loosens joints
- Improves joint mobility (especially heat and friction movements)
- Helps in the breakdown of adhesions
- Massage improves the blood and lymph flow in the muscles, which leads to better circulation in the underlying bones, benefiting their nutrition and growth

The urinary system

> **REMEMBER**
> The three types of postural deformities are kyphosis, scoliosis and lordosis.

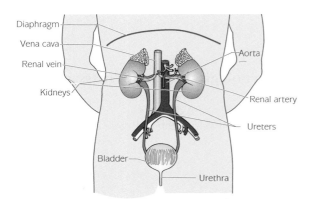

Diaphragm
Vena cava
Renal vein
Kidneys
Aorta
Renal artery
Ureters
Bladder
Urethra

Fig. 4.32 *The urinary system*

The urinary system filters blood and produces urine. It consists of two kidneys, two ureters, one urinary bladder and a single urethra. In metabolising nutrients, body cells produce wastes – carbon dioxide, excess water and heat. Several organs contribute to the job of waste elimination from the body.

The kidneys are located in the abdominal cavity. The right kidney is just below the liver and the left kidney below the spleen. The production of urine is made from the components of the kidneys, the nephrons.

There are three major functions/processes involved in the urinary system:

1. Filtration
2. Re-absorption
3. Secretion

The regulation of the urine production involves hormonal mechanisms (aldosterone) and nervous system stimulation.

Kidneys excrete:
- Water
- Nitrogenous wastes from protein catabolism
- Some bacterial toxins
- Hydrogen
- Inorganic salts (electrolytes)
- Some heat and carbon dioxide

Lungs excrete:
- Carbon dioxide
- Heat
- Some water

Skin excretes:
- Heat
- Water
- Carbon dioxide
- Small quantities of salt and urea

Gastro-intestinal tract eliminates:
- Solid undigested wastes

Excretes:
- Carbon dioxide
- Water
- Salts
- Heat

The physiological and psychological effects of massage on the urinary system
- Increases production of urine (lymph drainage)
- Promotes the activity of the kidneys which helps with the elimination of waste
- Reduces fluid retention
- Increases cell metabolism and expels additional carbon dioxide
- The use of abdominal and lower back massage promotes the activity of the kidneys which enhances the elimination of waste

Diseases and disorders of the urinary system include:
Cystisis
Kidney stones
Nephritis or Bright's disease
Urinary incontinence

1. List three main differences between arteries and veins.
2. Name three benefits of massage to the digestive system.
3. Name five endocrine glands found in the body and state their functions.
4. State five effects of massage on the skin.
5. What are the three stages of hair growth.
6. State three effects of massage on the lymphatic system.
7. List the three types of muscle found in the body.
8. Which parts make up the central nervous system.
9. State three effects massage has on the respiratory system.
10. Name the bones that make up the spine. How many bones make up each region?

Key Terms

You need to know what these words mean. Go back through the chapter or check in the glossary to find out.

- Cells
- Homeostasis
- Red blood cells
- White blood cells
- Platelets
- Arteries
- Veins
- Capillaries
- Pulse
- Digestion
- Pituitary gland
- Thyroid gland
- Parathyroid gland
- Adrenal gland
- Testes
- Ovaries
- Epidermis
- Dermis
- Lanugo
- Vellus
- Terminal
- Anagen
- Catogen
- Telogen
- Adipose tissue
- Lymphatic node

- Lymphatic vessel
- Lymph
- Involuntary muscle
- Voluntary muscle
- Cardiac muscle
- Central nervous system
- Peripheral nervous system
- Appendicular skeleton
- Axial skeleton

Prevention versus Cure

After working through this chapter you will be able to:
- have a deeper understanding of how IHM works
- identify conditions that could benefit from IHM.

The massage industry is peer regulated by several groups of therapists, with little government control or regulation. The industry is hugely disadvantaged by the fact that massage is often used as a cover for the sex industry. This has given rise to remedial body work centres with names where the word 'massage' is not used.

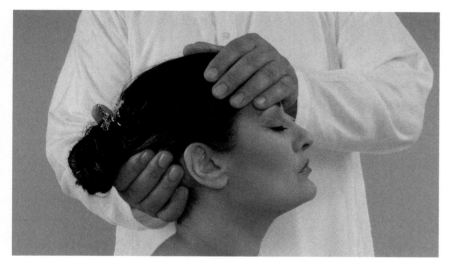

Fig. 5.01 *Receiving an Indian Head Massage*

As a definition, massage is any method of rubbing, stroking and therapeutic touch applied to the body. Massage is the refinement of our basic human instinct that, if it hurts, we rub it better. Anyone who has received any massage, even if only sincerely performed, receives the benefits of relaxation and a sense of greater wellbeing.

Ayurveda is an extremely precise, systematic and logical system that understands that the qualities of an item can become Ayurvedic. A food product from your back yard can become an Ayurvedic food if you understand and use the Ayurvedic system. In this way it is important to understand that Ayurveda is a way to perceive the world, not a product.

> **REMEMBER**
> Massage is any method of rubbing, stroking and therapeutic touch applied to the body.

Ayurveda can and must be adapted to the Western mind, environment and diet. If this is not done, it is a disservice to the system as a whole. While more and more therapists/practitioners are beginning to appear in the West, it is important to verify the tradition and training that a practitioner has had. It is also helpful to understand that a doctor of Ayurvedic medicine is different from a practitioner of Ayurveda. Choosing a health care professional is ultimately a question of personal preferences once this distinction is clear. The deeper secrets of Ayurveda are not necessarily learned – like life, they are experienced.

How Indian Head Massage works

It is generally assumed that the skull is a motionless piece of bone that does nothing but house the brain. On the contrary, the skull acts like a pump made up of many moving parts, separate plates of bone that move against each other. Each time you breathe in, your skull expands outward at the sides and downward at the top. When you breathe out, your skull comes in at the sides and up at the top. Its job is to promote the circulation of cerebro-spinal fluid that feeds distant nerves all over the body.

The expanding and contracting motion of the skull also increases the circulation of blood to the pituitary and to the rest of the brain. In addition, the skull 'pump' changes blood-flow patterns inside the brain. Regrettably many pressures are exerted on the skull which can compress the plates against each other in ways that compromise the brain's functioning. This can occur in childbirth or as a result of trauma later in life. Movement of skull plates is essential to life. Loss of motion can promote degenerative disease.

Organs represented in the scalp

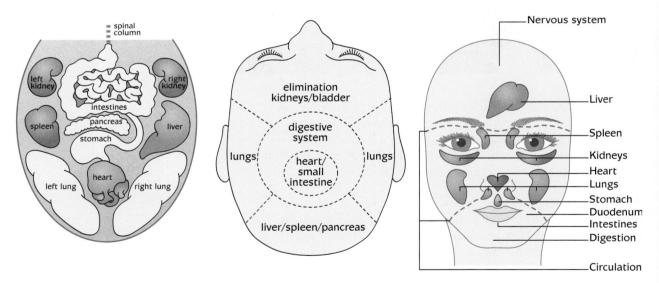

Fig. 5.02 *Organs represented in the scalp, face and tongue*

The head is very much like the ears, tongue, face, nails and feet in that it reflects other parts of the body.

- Massage at the centre crown of the scalp relates to the heart and small intestine
- As you spread out from the centre you approach the digestive system
- To the left and right above the ears in the temple areas, you have the lungs
- To the back of the head you have the liver, spleen and pancreas
- At the front of the skull you have the elimination of kidneys and bladder

For example: a red upper forehead appears if client's circulatory functions are overworked, causing a fast pulse. Overactive excretory functions can result in frequent urination and diarrhoea. White patches can mean over-consumption of dairy products, while over-consumption of sugar results in dark-coloured patches which can increase the risk of kidney stones and bladder infections.

Professional diagnostic skills not only reveal the presence of existing disorders but can also detect potential problems before they arise. This syllabus does not however qualify you to diagnose any medical conditions.

Ayurveda is not an endless repetition of curries and rigid Yogic practices. It is simply a very ancient, practical method to understand life. Ayurveda begins by helping each person understand themselves and their unique nature. Then it helps one to learn how diet, lifestyle, career, family and environment interact with our nature, causing balance or imbalance, health or disease, joy or sorrow. Ayurveda is a way to understand nature in precise detail or in broad generalities. Ayurveda is an open door to health.

> **REMEMBER**
> Ayurveda is a very ancient, practical method of understanding life.

It derived in ancient societies from the essentially spiritualistic transfer of a life force of healing power from divine healers and shamans to the sick, metamorphosing in time into the art of physical, restorative power by massage.

There is a detailed consultation form to be completed as well as a list of contraindications a therapist has to take into account. Indian Head Massage is a full treatment in its own right and should not be blended with another therapy, or curtailed.

What is the purpose of giving a massage?
- To strengthen the body?
- To help liberate toxins?
- To relax?
- To release tension?
- To maintain the three humours?
- To nourish the muscle and fat tissues?
- To open and release deep connections and feelings?
- Are you using massage as part of a strengthening programme?

The human touch is one of the surest ways of unburdening stresses. Just as the embrace of a parent soothes the upset child, just as a kiss or handshake takes the sting out of an argument, the simplest touch sometimes works miracles.

> **REMEMBER**
> The simplest touch sometimes works miracles.

The healing process

Acting Ayurveda – Shalyakya Tantra

Shalyakya Tantra is one of the eight branches of the Ayurvedic treatment tree. This branch is dedicated to the treatment of diseases located above the neck. Chalky Tantra actually covers the treatment part of pathologies above the neck. It accounts for all types of problems in and around the head. This is done by applying medication, with the help of probes, to the affected part.

Shalyakya Tantra is described in detail in the books *Sushrut Sanhita, Charak Sanhita* and *Ashtang Hruday* (literally meaning the heart of the eight-branched body of Ayurveda)

The name Shalyakya Tantra has arrived from the word 'Shalaka', meaning probe. Different types of probes are available with Ayurvedic treatment. These include:

- Probe of the eye – netra shalaka
- Probe of the ear – karna shalaka
- Probe of the nose – nasa shalaka
- Probe of the throat – mukh shalaka
- Probe of the lips – oshta shalaka

Shalyakya Tantra has listed about 72 diseases of the eye (netra rog) including conjunctivitis (sarvakshi rog), cataract (linganash), pre-glaucomatic condition and glaucoma (timir) and diseases of the iris/pupil (drushti rog). In addition, it has listed:

25 diseases of the ear – karna rog
18 diseases of the nose – nasa rog
11 diseases of the lips – oshta rog
1 disease of the lymph glands – gand rog
23 diseases of the teeth – danta rog
6 diseases of the tongue – jiva rog
8 diseases of the palate – talu rog
18 diseases of the throat-pharynx-larynx – gal rog
8 diseases of the oral cavity – sarvagat mukhrog

Follow-up treatment for all the above-mentioned problems are also precisely described.

When Ayurveda entered the history of mankind, anaesthesia was not around, nor septic precautions. But Ayurvedic sages described ashchotananjan-vidhi (putting Ayurvedic medicinal drops in the eyes) and putpak-vidhi (covering the eye with a smooth medicated cloth or tree leaf) to avoid spreading infections.

The first surgeon in the history of Ayurvedic medicine named Sushruta says putpak-vidhi is equally important and covers half of the aspect of ophthalmologic treatment. A stipulated therapy that includes all these procedures, step by step, is discussed in detail in the *Sushrut Sanhita*.

In addition to this, surgical intervention for tumours, abscesses and cysts (arbuda), and attempts to remove foreign bodies in the region above the neck are listed in the Shalyakya Tantra. Etiology, diagnosis and treatment of diseases of the eye, ear, nose and throat, and oral cavity are covered in the Shalyakya Tantra. Migraine (ardha-shishi) is also included in Shalyakya Tantra with a change in lifestyle recommended for its prevention and cure.

This Ayurvedic branch of medicine and surgery related to problems of the region above the neck has also suggested some simple remedies for day-to-day problems like dryness of the eyes, ear, nose, and throat, and oral cavity.

This clearly suggests that Ayurveda was a science meant not only for advanced diseases, but for common health problems as well.

Elements from the therapist's fingers are attracted to certain organs in the client.

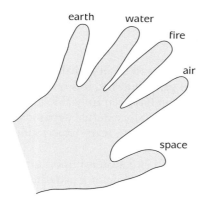

earth   water   fire   air   space

Fig. 5.03 *Palmplan*

Your fingerprints are unique; everything you touch and feel in this world will carry your signature.

The body possesses the innate ability to heal itself. Healing works on the principle that increasing the prana or life force in the affected part of the physical body accelerates the healing process.

Healing through touch influences this natural life force to bring about a healthier physical body when applied to the electromagnetic field known as the aura, which contains the mould and blueprint of the physical body.

This bioplasmic body absorbs life energy and distributes it to the organs and glands. Diseases first appear as energetic disruptions in the energy field before presenting as ailments in the physical body.

Healing through Shiro-Abhyanga's unique matrix of prana-chakra-nadi-marma realigns the whole energy system to help initiate specific biochemical changes which accelerate the body's natural ability to prevent and alleviate a wide spectrum of physical, emotional and psychological ailments.

Jiva
The Jiva is the organ of taste and speech. We perceive taste through the tongue when it is wet; a dry tongue cannot perceive taste. The tongue is also used to convey words, thoughts, concepts, ideas and feelings.

Different parts of the tongue are related to different organs in the body. If there are discolourations, depressions or elevations in certain areas of the tongue, the respective organs are defective. For example, the coating covering the tongue relates to toxins in small/large intestines.

Neem tree twigs are traditionally chewed, then used as a toothbrush and finally as a tongue cleaner. This application has been approved by researchers in Germany, who found the neem bark extracts were effective against tooth decay and periodontal disease, such as gingivitis.

Table 5.01

Whitish tongue	Kapa derangement
Red or yellow-green tongue	Pita derangement
Black-to-brown tongue	Vata derangement

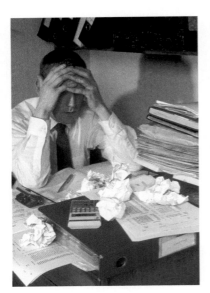

Fig. 5.04 *The effects of stress*

Stress

Stress is neither negative nor positive. It is our body's normal response to challenge, threat or excitement. The stress response is only a problem if it occurs too often, exists for too long before dissipating, or occurs with a force that is too strong.

The concept of stress is familiar to us all and although most people understand its meaning in general terms, it is often difficult to define precisely. No single definition has been fully able to describe the nature of stress. Stress is not only imposed by external demands but can also be generated from within, by our hopes, fears, expectations and beliefs.

Our individual judgement of a situation is important in initiating a stress response. If it is assessed as demanding or frustrating it will engender a physiological response with mental, emotional, physical and behavioural components.

Stress, then, is a specific response the body makes to various demands, for example being exposed to threat, or struggling to meet unrealistic expectations of others as well as our own. Whatever the situation is, when the demand we perceive exceeds the resources we think we have, the body and mind are aroused and all systems are geared up either to fight the challenge or to flee the challenge.

We all function with a certain amount of stress, however it is only when that level reaches an unsupportable limit that clients complain of too much stress or they produce stress symptoms.

- Too little stress indicates insufficient challenge, lack of stimulation and often boredom, indicating a lack of purpose or meaning in life.
- Optimum stress is where we seek to maintain a balanced life.
- Too much stress is a constant feeling of having too much to do. One is no longer able to take time off to rest and play. Performance drops through being in permanent overdrive.
- Breakdown is when an individual feels out of control and shows signs of physical and psychological breakdown. With excessive stress clients may come to rely on alcohol, smoking and tranquillizers or sleeping pills in order to blank out the stress. Accidents may occur and the client is often preoccupied with unresolved tension and may become withdrawn or aggressive.

If these signs are not heeded, ultimately the mind and body will break down, either physically or mentally, or both. We need to strike a balance. Life is not a short run, it is a marathon requiring us to take control of how we use our pranic resource so we do not deplete our reserves.

We often hear of sportspeople 'psyching themselves up' or 'getting their adrenalin flowing' before an important event, in order to improve their performance. These situations tell us something important about stress: it can either be a barrier or an aid to success depending on how you interpret, label and control it.

Indian Head Massage offers an instant de-stressing programme for the entire body. Physical benefits are obtained immediately with specific relaxation of the muscles and the easing of tension. Of particular value in the workplace are the benefits of relieving mental tiredness. Clearer thinking is promoted, leading to higher levels of alertness and concentration. Many clients describe the treatments as being almost sleep-inducing and afterwards report a wonderful feeling of wellbeing, lightness and being full of energy.

Massage can help with hyperactivity, heart ailments and circulatory disorders. It helps the body digest food and eliminate waste materials, stimulates the nervous and muscular systems, and aids the circulation of blood. It encourages the toxins that gather in muscles to disperse. Massage promotes feelings of calmness and tranquillity and is excellent for depression and anxiety. Although a single massage will be enjoyable, the effects of massage are cumulative and a course of massage treatments will bring the most benefits.

REMEMBER
Indian Head Massage offers an instant de-stressing programme for the entire body.

REMEMBER
Massage promotes feelings of calmness and tranquillity.

REMEMBER
Endorphins released from the brain help to elevate the mood.

Table 5.02 *Effects of stress on bodily functions*

Body part	Normal/relaxed	Under pressure
Brain	Blood supply normal	Blood supply increase
Mood	Happy	Serious
Saliva	Normal	Reduced
Muscles	Blood supply normal	Blood supply increase
Heart	Normal heart rate and blood pressure	Output rate and blood pressure increase
Lungs	Normal respiration	Respiration rate increase
Stomach	Normal blood supply and acid secretion	Blood supply decrease and acid secretion increase
Bowels	Normal blood supply and activity	Blood supply decrease and motility increase
Bladder	Normal function	Frequent micturition
Sexual organs	(M) normal sex (F) normal period, etc.	(M) impotence (blood supply decreases) (F) irregular periods
Skin	Healthy	Dry skin, blood supply decreases
Biochemistry	Normal oxygen consumed, glucose and fats liberated	Oxygen consumption increases, glucose and fat utilisation increases

Table 5.03 *Effects and benefits of massage*

Effects	Benefits
Increase in blood flow to the head, arms, neck and shoulder	• Improves circulation. The delivery of oxygen and nutrients is improved via the arterial circulation, and the removal of wastes is hastened via the venous flow • Brings more oxygen and nutrients into the muscles, reduces muscle fatigue and soreness • Increases sebum production helping to improve the skin's suppleness and resistance to infections • Increases production of sweat from sweat glands • Helps to temporarily decrease blood pressure due to dilation of capillaries • Vasodilatation of the surface capillaries helps to improve the skin's colour • Dilates blood vessels helping them to work more efficiently • Increases nutrition to the cells and encourages cell regeneration • Nourishes the tissues and encourages healing • Assists with excretion of urea and waste products through the skin • Improves elasticity of the skin • Reduces ischaemia
Massage deepens respiration and improves lung capacity	• Relaxes any tightness in the respiratory muscles
Strengthens the immune system	• Increases nutrition to white blood cells
Increases lymphatic flow to the head, neck and shoulders	• Stimulates immunity • Aids the elimination of accumulated toxins and waste products • Reduces oedema (excess fluid in the tissue) by increasing lymphatic drainage
Relaxes the muscles and nerves of fibres of the head, neck and shoulders	• Improves posture • Relieves muscular tension and fatigue • Can help to relieve tension headaches and aches and pains • Eases tightness, stiffness, spasms and restrictions allowing flexibility
Reduces spasms, restrictions and adhesions in the muscle fibres	• Relieves pain and discomfort • Improves joint mobility
Decreases inflammation in the tissues	• Pain relief • Reduces stress placed on the bones and joints
Calming or stimulation of the sympathetic nervous system	• Slows down the heart rate • Reduces stress and anxiety • Helps reduce blood pressure • Rejuvenates and boosts energy • Slows down and deepens breathing
Activates the parasympathetic nervous system	• Encourages the body to rest and relax • Promotes restful sleep
Improves circulation to the scalp	• Promotes healthy hair growth • Helps improve the condition of the skin and hair
Relaxes and soothes tense eye muscles	• Helps relieve tired eyes and eyestrain • Brightens the eyes
Increases the supply of oxygen to the brain	• Helps relieve mental fatigue • Promotes clearer thinking • Improves concentration • Increases productivity

Table 5.03 *Continued*

Effects	Benefits
Stimulates the release of endorphins, the brain's natural opiates	• Generates confidence and a feeling of wellbeing • Elevates the mood – can help anxiety and depression • Helps relieve emotional stress and repressed feelings • Helps relieve pain
Encourages the release of stagnant energy flow	• Creates a feeling of balance and calm
Enhances the awareness of breathing in one's own body therefore improves posture	• Helps to improve nutrients to soft tissues and joints • Helps to improve drainage of waste products and toxic substances away from congested areas • Helps to lengthen compressed joints • Improves posture
Helps loosen stiff joints and encourages movement where it is deficient	• Reduces any thickening of the connective tissue and helps to release restrictions in the facia • Helps to free adhesions, break down scar tissue and decrease inflammation • Reduces the physical stress in joints and bones
Can increase peristalsis in the large intestine	• Helps to relieve constipation, colic and wind and promote the activity of the para-sympathetic nervous system, which stimulates digestion
Increases urinary output	• Increases circulation and lymph drainage from the tissues
Promotes feeling of wellbeing	• Physically revitalising • Enhances self-esteem • Promotes positive body awareness and an improved body image through relaxation • Eases emotional trauma through relaxation • Reduces stress and anxiety by relaxing both the mind and body
Psychological benefits	• Antidote to stress, depression, anxiety and mental tension • Clears mind and revitalises mental capacity thus improving alertness and concentration levels • Provides support to all levels of holistic healing • Encourages a sense of calmness and serenity • Works on balancing chakras by releasing stagnant prana • Decongests and detoxifies • Rebalances body rhythms • Provides lasting benefit • Alleviates pain

Conditions where Indian Head Massage treatment has been used

Indian Head Massage treatments have been used as part of an allopathic health service programme, where it has the potential to stimulate the body to heal itself. It can be used as part of a client's relaxation routine and may also have the potential to combat the side effects of certain necessary drug regimes.

GOOD PRACTICE

Indian Head Massage is complementary to allopathic medicine.

Acne

An inflammatory disease of the sebaceous glands and hair follicles of the skin, that is marked by the eruption of pimples or pustules, especially on the face.

Addictions

The condition of being habitually or compulsively occupied with or involved in something; the compulsive physiological and psychological need for a habit-forming substance such as drugs or alcohol.

AIDS/HIV

HIV (Human Immunodeficiency Virus) is a retrovirus that infects cells of the human immune system. It is widely accepted that infection with HIV causes Acquired Immunodeficiency Syndrome (AIDS), a disease characterised by the destruction of the immune system.

Allergies

An allergy, or Type I hypersensitivity, is an immune malfunction whereby a person's body is hyper-sensitised to react to typically non-reactive substances.

Amenorrhoea

The absence of a menstrual period in a woman of reproductive age.

Amnesia

A condition in which memory is disturbed. The causes of amnesia are organic or functional. Organic causes include damage to the brain, through trauma or disease, or use of certain (generally sedative) drugs. Functional causes are psychological factors, such as defence mechanisms.

Angina

Chest discomfort usually described as pressure, heaviness, squeezing, burning or a choking sensation. Angina is usually precipitated by exertion or emotional stress, and exacerbated by having a full stomach or by cold temperatures.

Anorexia

The symptom of diminished appetite or appetite loss. The eating disorder anorexia nervosa is commonly referred to simply as anorexia. Common disorders that cause anorexia include anorexia nervosa, severe depression, cancer, dementia, AIDS and chronic renal disease.

Anxiety

Anxiety is part of the 'fight or flight' response to stress, which is an adaptive response to danger in the environment. The symptoms are irritability, inability to concentrate, sleep problems, overactive mind, breathlessness, aches and pains, nausea, dry mouth and changes in appetite. Rarely, it can lead to more pronounced symptoms such as panic attacks. Stress plays an important role that can be linked to genetics, personality type, bad experiences and family behaviour patterns.

Arthritis

Arthritic diseases include rheumatoid arthritis and prosaic arthritis, which are auto-immune diseases; septic arthritis, caused by joint infection; and the more common osteo-arthritis, or degenerative joint disease. Arthritis

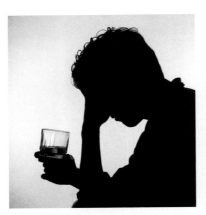

Fig. 5.05 *Alcohol addiction*

> **REMEMBER**
> Indian head massage can form part of an effective treatment for someone who has an anxiety disorder.

can be caused by strains and injuries from repetitive motion, sports, overexertion and falls.

Asthma
Asthma is a complex disease characterised by bronchial hyper-responsiveness (BHR), inflammation and intermittent airway obstruction. A person with asthma may experience wheezing, shortness of breath, chest tightness and cough, particularly after exposure to an allergen, cold air, exercise, or when emotional.

Auto-immune diseases
Arise from an overactive immune response of the body against substances and tissues normally present in the body. There are more than 40 human diseases classified as auto-immune diseases; almost all appear without warning or apparent cause.

Some examples of auto-immune diseases are: Crohn's disease, lupus erythematosus, multiple sclerosis, psoriasis, Grave's disease and diabetes mellitus (type 1).

Baldness
Hair reflects our inner health and can be affected by our lifestyle, the foods we eat and stress. Hair loss in men is related to hormone levels and pattern of heredity – although it is normal in older men. Severe stress and shock can also contribute. Hair loss in women can result from dietary deficiencies or hormonal imbalances – it can happen after pregnancy as hormone levels drop, in individuals suffering from anorexia, or in women who are suffering from hypothyroidism.

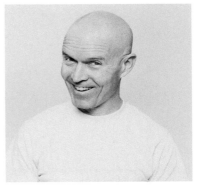

Fig. 5.06 *Male pattern baldness*

Bell's palsy
Bell's palsy is a disorder of the facial nerve, which controls the muscles of the upper and middle areas of the face. It often results from a previous viral infection in which the nerve becomes damaged. Typical symptoms result from the paralysis of the muscles served by the nerve. These include sagging of the mouth, dribbling, impairment of taste, and watering or dryness of the eye on the affected side of the head. On examination, the Bell's palsy sufferer is typically unable to wrinkle their forehead, close their eyes tightly, or whistle or blow out of their cheeks.

Body odour
Is the result of perspiration and whatever bacteria are growing on the body. Odour can be influenced by diet, gender, heredity, health, medications, occupation and mood. Generally body odour is associated with the hair, skin, breasts, armpits and genitals.

Bulimia
An eating disorder where the person engages in recurrent binge eating followed by one or more of the following: vomiting, inappropriate use of laxatives, enemas, diuretics, excessive exercising or fasting.

Cancer
Cancer is not one disease. It is a group of more than 100 different and distinctive diseases. Cancer develops from a single cell that has undergone mutations in its deoxyribonucleic acid (DNA). Instead of maturing normally and dying, cancerous cells reproduce without restraint – they proliferate in an uncontrolled way and, in some cases, metastasise (spread).

Skin cancer is the most common type of malignancy for both men and women; the second most common type in men is prostate cancer, and in women, breast cancer.

Carpal tunnel syndrome
A painful progressive condition caused by compression of the median nerve in the wrist. Symptoms are pain, weakness or numbness in the hand and wrist, radiating up the arm. Commonly occurs in those performing repetitive work.

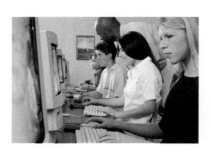

Fig. 5.07 *Computer usage – a common cause of RSI*

Repetitive strain injuries (RSI) occur from repeated physical movements doing damage to tendons, nerves, muscles and other soft body tissues. Occupations ranging from musicians to computer operators have characteristic RSI. The rise of computer use and flat, light-touch keyboards that permit high-speed typing has resulted in an epidemic of injuries of the hands, arms and shoulders.

Cerebral palsy
Cerebral palsy is a contractible disease or illness which is not contagious and can affect anybody. Cerebral palsy is a physically disabling neurological condition, which affects the physical and mental parts of the human body. Somebody who suffers from cerebral palsy needs constant care throughout their life, as in most cases they have severe difficulty in walking, talking and therefore caring for themselves.

Chronic fatigue syndrome
Prolonged fatigue can be a symptom of a number of conditions, including anaemia, depression, chronic infection, candida, auto-immune disorder and cancer. For some kinds of extreme fatigue, however, no apparent cause can be found, even though the problem may persist for years. Complementary practitioners are more ready to look beyond the symptoms for possible contributing factors. This increasingly common condition has acquired various names, although the most generally accepted is chronic fatigue syndrome. It is also known as ME in the UK.

> **REMEMBER**
> Chronic fatigue syndrome is also known as ME in the UK.

Colitis
Colitis is a disease almost exclusively of civilised nations – put in the class of ailments called 'civilised diseases'. This stems from its main causes, which are dietary, and lifestyle in origin – a refined diet, sedentary lifestyle and stress. The symptoms of chronic colitis are: abdominal pain, abdominal distension, cramps, wind, constipation, diarrhoea and mucus.

Concentration
The cognitive process of giving selective attention to one thing while ignoring other things.

Constipation
Constipation is the infrequent and difficult passing of small hard stools. It can cause piles and fissures and other painful problems. If it is an ongoing problem it can lead to a coated tongue, halitosis, lack of energy and mental dullness.

> **REMEMBER**
> Simple lifestyle re-adjustments can help to cure constipation: a high-fibre diet, plenty of fluid intake, daily exercise and learning a relaxation technique.

The causes of constipation are commonly a low-fibre diet, insufficient fluid intake, a sedentary lifestyle, although stress, habitual use of laxatives, pregnancy and ageing can cause the condition. It is also a symptom of irritable bowel syndrome.

Cramps

An unpleasant sensation caused by contraction, usually of a muscle. Can be caused by cold or over-exertion, illness or poisoning.

Crohn's disease

A chronic inflammation of the digestive tract, particularly the lower small intestine. It is mainly a disease of Western civilisation and occurs most often in people aged 15 to 35. The symptoms are pain, bloating, fever, fatigue, weight loss and vitamin and mineral deficiencies. The joints, eyes and skin might also become inflamed.

Some believe Crohn's disease may be caused by lifestyle factors such as refined diet, lack of exercise and stress. Others, however, think that it may be an auto-immune response, particularly as the intestines are sensitive to stress. There is some evidence that it might be genetic as it runs in families.

Dandruff

Dandruff occurs as fine white scales flaking from the scalp. It is often a result of seborrhoeic eczema, but it can be related to psoriasis or caused by a fungal infection – in this case it is thought it might be related to the fungus candida albicans. Dandruff is extremely common and not serious. Conventionally it is treated with medicated shampoo – although complementary treatments are more likely to favour a systemic approach as it may merely be caused by a dry scalp.

Dementia

A progressive decline in cognitive function, in particular affecting memory, attention, language, motor skills and problem solving. Subject may appear disoriented and depressed.

Depression

Most people experience some form of depression at some point in their lives. The depression is used to describe a range of negative feelings from mild, temporary down feelings, to clinical or major depression.

The causes of depression are complex and can include: worries related to finances, work and health, relationship problems and bereavement. Depression can be triggered by the hormonal changes which occur at different life stages such as in puberty, menstruation and after giving birth (post-natal depression). Depression can sometimes arise from the physiological changes that result from organic disease. Re-living distressing or traumatic events, as in post-traumatic stress disorder, can also trigger depression.

In addition, some personalities seem more vulnerable. The symptoms of depression can be both physical and mental and include: disturbed sleep patterns and appetite disturbance, mood swings, restlessness, tearfulness, inability to concentrate, impatience, aggression, loss of interest in everyday activities and in the most severe cases feelings of hopelessness, excessive guilt, despair and suicide.

Diabetes (mellitus)

An auto-immune disease caused by decreased production of insulin by the pancreas. Requires insulin injections to keep blood-sugar levels within normal limits to prevent complications such as cardiovascular disease, chronic renal failure and retinal damage.

REMEMBER
Re-living distressing or traumatic events, as in post-traumatic stress disorder, can trigger depression.

- Diabetes Type 1
  Develops when the insulin-producing cell in the pancreas has been destroyed, so the body can no longer produce any insulin

- Diabetes Type 2
  Develops when the body can still produce some insulin but not enough to keep blood-sugar level stable, or the body can't use it effectively

Diarrhoea

A condition which is a symptom of disease, food-borne illness or injury. Is usually accompanied by abdominal pain and often vomiting or nausea. Usually caused by viral infections but can also be caused by bacterial toxins and infection.

Drugs

A substance used in the diagnosis, treatment or prevention of a disease or as a component of a medication.

Dysmenorrhoea (menstruation)

Normal menstruation that is painful is known as primary dysmenorrhoea, while secondary dysmenorrhoea refers to period pain caused by reproductive disorders such as endometriosis. In primary dysmenorrhoea it is thought that the muscles of the uterus squeeze and contract harder than normal to dislodge the thickened lining. These contractions may also hamper blood flow to the uterus, exacerbating the pain. Women of any age can experience painful periods and some women find that periods are no longer painful after pregnancy and childbirth.

Dysmenorrhoea can be associated with: headache, nausea and vomiting, digestive upsets, such as diarrhoea or constipation, fainting, and pre-menstrual symptoms, such as tender breasts and swollen abdomen, which may continue throughout the period.

Dyspepsia

Disturbed digestion, indigestion. A constant pain in the stomach. Can be caused by stomach ulcers or aggravated by high acidity in the stomach.

Eating disorders

An eating disorder is a syndrome in which a person eats in a way which disturbs their physical health. Overeating is the most common and obvious such disorder. Other major recognised eating disorders are anorexia nervosa, bulimia nervosa and binge-eating disorder. People whose eating is disordered in these ways experience psychological suffering, typically becoming obsessed with food, diet and body image. Their health is at extreme risk due to malnutrition.

Eczema

An inflammatory condition of the skin, which appears as redness, itching and oozing lesions, which can become scaly, crusted or hardened.

Endometriosis

Occurs when endometrial tissue locates and grows in places other than the uterus. Results in severe pain and can lead to infertility.

Enuresis
Incontinence; involuntary discharge of urine.

Epilepsy
Refers to a number of disorders caused by abnormal electrical discharges in the brain. Characterised by sudden and often brief instances of altered or diminished consciousness, involuntary movements and/or convulsions.

Exam stress
Test-taking anxiety or stress is very common among the student population. It can be very distressing and sometimes debilitating. Often students find they get good course grades, but that their grades drop in exams.

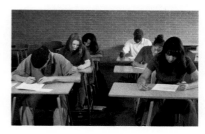
Fig. 5.08 *Exam-taking can cause stress*

Fatigue
Physical or mental weariness resulting from exertion or stress.

Fibromyalgia
A chronic disorder characterised by widespread musculo-skeletal pain, fatigue, and multiple tender areas that occur in localised regions, particularly the neck, shoulders, spine and hips. Clients with this syndrome may also experience sleep disturbances, morning stiffness, irritable bowel syndrome, anxiety and other symptoms.

Frigidity
Persistent aversion to sexual intercourse.

Glandular disorders
A disorder of the glands of the body.

Gout
A metabolic disturbance caused by elevated levels of uric acid in the blood and deposits of urate crystals around the joints. Characterised by painful inflammation of the joints, especially the feet and hands. Can become chronic.

Halitosis
The condition of having foul-smelling breath.

Hay fever
An allergic reactionary condition caused by an abnormal sensitivity to airborne pollen. Most often characterised by sneezing, itchy, watery eyes, and nasal discharge and congestion.

Headaches and migraines
Headaches can range in severity from dull thudding in the temples when you are tired or anxious, to a frightening, intense pain. Lifestyle factors, musculo-skeletal disorders or stress may trigger them and it is important to find and remedy the underlying causes. One of the most common symptoms of stress is the tension headache, mainly caused by tension in the muscles of the face, scalp, neck and back.

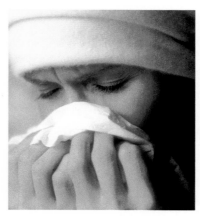
Fig. 5.09 *A hay fever sufferer*

Migraines affect at least one person in ten and are far more disabling then headaches. They are often confined to one side of the head and may be preceded or accompanied by visual disturbances, e.g. flashing lights or hallucinatory auras, pins and needles, nausea and sensitivity to odours, light or noise.

REMEMBER
Backache can also be a
result of tension in muscles.

Migraines tend to run in families and can be triggered by the same factors that cause headaches or by sensitivity to particular substances. Migraines can also be brought on by stress. These are caused by spasms occurring in the blood vessels that supply the brain.

Hormone replacement therapy (HRT)

The administration of oestrogen and progesterone to relieve the symptoms of the menopause. It reduces the risk of heart disease and can prevent osteoporosis in post-menopausal women.

Hyper and hypo activity of the pituitary gland

The pituitary gland is a small oval endocrine organ attached to the base of the brain. It produces various hormones, which directly or indirectly affect most basic bodily functions by controlling or influencing other endocrine organs. Hyperactive pituitary (acromegaly) is usually caused by a tumour and can result in gigantism when it occurs in children, or disproportionate thickening of bones in adults, due to hypersecretion of growth hormone. Frequently, glucose metabolism is disturbed leading to diabetes mellitus. Hypoactive pituitary disorders cause various disturbances depending on which hormone is being produced insufficiently. Common disorders include hypothyroidism, underactive adrenal glands, and stunted growth or dwarfism in children.

Hyperactive thyroid

A condition caused by the thyroid producing too much thyroid hormone. Common symptoms include palpitations, heat intolerance, nervousness, insomnia, breathlessness, increased bowel movements, light or absent menstrual periods, and fatigue.

Hypothyroidism

A condition where the thyroid does not produce enough thyroid hormone. It is considered to be an auto-immune disorder. Can be caused by the pituitary not producing enough thyroid stimulating hormone (TSH). Symptoms are fatigue, weakness, weight gain or difficulty losing weight, coarse, dry hair, dry, rough skin, hair loss, cold intolerance, muscle cramps and aches, constipation, depression, irritability, memory loss, abnormal menstrual cycles, decreased libido.

Impotence (erectile dysfunction)

A failure to have or maintain a penis erection due to physical or psychological causes.

Incontinence

The inability to control excretory functions.

Indigestion

Indigestion is an umbrella term for discomfort of the upper abdomen or stomach, usually after eating. It is also known as dyspepsia or acid stomach. Symptoms include heartburn, belching, hiccups, nausea and flatulence. Persistent problems with indigestion may be due to a peptic ulcer or liver, gall bladder or pancreatic disease.

The causes of indigestion range from indulging in too much rich, spicy or fatty food, excess alcohol, eating too quickly and eating unripe fruit. Pregnant women can suffer from indigestion because their intestines are

REMEMBER
Stress, anxiety and
unresolved emotions can
cause indigestion.

pushed up into the thoracic cavity causing reflux (acid flowing back into the oesophagus).

Insomnia

Insomnia is defined as difficulty in falling asleep, waking frequently or waking from sleep prematurely with difficulty in returning to sleep.

A minimum amount of sleep is needed for many body functions; too little can lead to irritability, depression, digestive problems, emotional disturbances and poor memory.

The causes of insomnia are varied, but most common is psychological. Trouble in falling asleep is associated with anxiety; difficulty in remaining asleep is linked to depression, illness, persistent pain or changes to the daily body clock. Lack of exercise, stimulants such as caffeine, nicotine, alcohol or change in sleep surroundings can affect sleep rhythms.

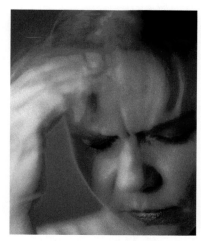

Fig. 5.10 *Insomnia is linked to anxiety*

Irritable bowel syndrome (IBS)

IBS is also known as spastic or irritable colon. It is the most common gastro-intestinal complaint, affecting one in ten people. It is characterised by abdominal pain, constipation, diarrhoea, cramps, abdominal distension, excessive wind, and lethargy. IBS appears to be brought on and exacerbated by anxiety, stress and nervous problems.

Symptoms often appear worse during menstruation and indeed IBS seems to occur more in women. Other causal factors include food intolerance, a diet that is too high in refined carbohydrates, caffeine or sugar, and a sedentary lifestyle.

Leucorrhoea

A thick, whitish discharge from the vagina or cervical canal.

Low motility

Refers to a low percentage of sperm that move or 'swim'. Typically, 50% swimmers are considered normal. The more moving sperm that are present, the more likely they are to successfully inseminate an egg. It is believed that smoking, excessive alcohol and caffeine use, excessive stress, excessive heat to the scrotum, and toxic chemicals can all adversely affect sperm motility.

Low sperm count

Causes of male infertility can be either temporary or permanent. Temporary causes include heavy-duty cycling, exposure to extreme heat, ill-fitting briefs and emotional stress. Substance abuse, smoking, malnutrition, obesity, genetic factors, radiation treatments and environmental assaults can all affect sperm count permanently. Regular exercise, relaxation exercises, maintaining a healthy weight, and avoiding exposure to heavy metal toxins can all help to correct this condition.

Lung disease

High stress levels are associated with increased incidence of smoking which can influence the onset of pneumonia, influenza and emphysema. Stress has been shown to have a very direct link with asthma. In a widespread investigation conducted by Melhuish (1978), emotional factors were found to be relevant in 70% of asthmatic patients studied.

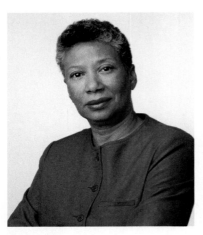

Fig. 5.11 *Menopause usually occurs between the ages of 45 and 55*

Lupus

An auto-immune disorder in which antibodies are created against the subject's own deoxyribonucleic acid (DNA). Patients may have thick red scaly patches on the skin in the shape of a butterfly. Usually causes joint pain often in the hand and wrist. Can result in anaemia and iron deficiency, and inflammation of various parts of the heart.

Menopause

Occurs when the ovaries naturally stop producing oestrogen, which causes the cessation of menstruation. Menopause usually occurs between the ages of 45 and 55.

Morning sickness

Nausea and vomiting that occurs during pregnancy commonly starting in the first month and continuing until the 14th or 16th week.

Motor neurone disease (MND)

MND is caused by the degeneration of the nerves in the central nervous system. It is characterised by weakness and wasting of the muscles, leading to uncontrolled muscle spasms and stiffness. Ultimately, breathing and swallowing are affected. Some alternative therapies can help to ease symptoms – although nerve degeneration cannot be controlled.

Mucus colon

Healthy mucus in the colon contains a large volume of alkaline-buffering agents which protect the bowel wall from acids and toxins. Abnormal build-up of mucus, however, has been associated with pathogenic bacteria and bowel disease. Excessive stress, ingesting meat and milk products, as well as misuse of drugs, alcohol and salt can disrupt the normal healthy pH of our digestive systems and contribute to the increase in unhealthy mucins.

Multiple sclerosis (MS)

MS is a progressive degenerative disease that occurs when the myelin sheath (the protective fatty tissue enveloping nerves) becomes inflamed. The myelin sheath is not only protective but is also involved in message transmission along the nerve. The inflammation therefore results in a number of nerve problems. Symptoms include blurred vision and slurred speech and motor neurone difficulties, including loss of co-ordination and paralysis. This can lead to bladder, mental, emotional, speech and sexual problems.

Muscular dystrophy

A group of hereditary diseases characterised by progressive skeletal muscle weakness. Can appear in infancy, childhood or adulthood.

Myalgic encephalomyelitis (ME) (chronic fatigue syndrome)

A potentially disabling and chronic condition affecting the immune and central nervous system. Characterised by exercise-induced muscle fatigue, muscle pain, and flu-like malaise, sore throat, swollen glands and poor concentration and memory.

Myasthenia gravis

This term literally means grave muscle weakness. It is a chronic auto-immune, neuromuscular disease characterised by varying degrees of weakness of the skeletal muscles of the body. The symptoms are seen to increase during periods of activity, and improve with rest. Often affects the muscles controlling eye and eyelid movement and facial muscles.

Non-specific infertility
Inability to conceive with no apparent cause.

Ovarian cysts
A cyst is a fluid-filled sac. A cyst is formed on the ovary each month during a normal menstrual cycle. Occasionally, these sacs close off after their cycle and continue to collect fluid and grow. This condition can result in bleeding or can twist the ovary and cause pain.

Pain management
Acute and chronic pain is commonly managed in a variety of ways including pharmacologically – using analgesics and narcotics; non-pharmacologically – such as ice or heat or massage; or psychologically – such as with cognitive therapy or biofeedback methods.

Panic attack
An episode of intense fear or apprehension characterised by four or more symptoms – sensations of choking, heart palpitations, dizziness, shortness of breath, trembling, nausea, dizziness, hyperventilation and/or tingling sensations. Panic attacks come on suddenly, appear to be unprovoked and are often disabling.

Parkinson's disease
A neuro-degenerative disease which occurs when the neurones in the part of the brain called the substantia nigra die or become impaired. These neurones normally produce dopamine, which allows for the smooth, co-ordinated functions of the body's muscles and movement. Key signs of Parkinson's disease are: tremors, slowness of movement, rigidity (stiffness) and difficulty with balance, stiff facial expressions, shuffling walk, muffled speech and depression.

Peptic ulcers
Stomach ulcers or peptic ulcers are caused by the action of stomach acid on the lining of the mucous membranes of the stomach wall. Symptoms vary but can include: a localised growing burning pain, heartburn, local tenderness, nausea, vomiting and diarrhoea. The pain usually begins just after eating or within twenty minutes of a meal. Drinking, smoking, stress and taking aspirin may all contribute to the formation of an ulcer.

Pregnancy
It is normal to experience some minor discomfort during pregnancy. The most common reason for not feeling well, especially in the early months, is morning sickness – this is caused by an increase in hormone levels during the early months of pregnancy. It normally disappears by the third month. There may be other minor ailments such as sore breasts due to hormonal changes, and heartburn, which can occur during the final months of pregnancy when the abdomen is pushing up into the thoracic cavity.

Pre-menstrual syndrome (PMS)
A term used to cover a wide range of symptoms experienced by some women for up to two weeks before a monthly period. Typical symptoms

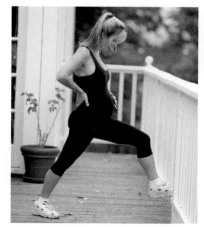

Fig. 5.12 *Minor discomfort can occur during pregnancy*

include: water retention, weight gain, headaches, swollen joints, depression, insomnia, irritability and poor concentration.

Prostate disorders

A large percentage of men over the age of fifty suffer from prostate problems. The main three are hypertrophy or enlargement of the prostate gland, prostatitis or inflammation in the prostate gland, and cancer of the prostate gland.

Psoriasis

A non-contagious, lifelong skin condition which appears as raised red patches or lesions, covered with a silvery-white build-up of dead skin cells, called scale. Psoriasis can occur on any part of the body and affects both men and women.

Recurrent cystitis

Characterised by at least two infections of the bladder in six months or three infections in one year. Symptoms are painful or burning urination, urinary frequency and urgency, and possibly blood in the urine.

Reproductive disorders

Disorders that may affect the proper functioning of the reproductive system include: abnormal hormone secretion, sexually transmitted diseases and other conditions that may affect fertility or complicate pregnancy.

Rheumatoid arthritis

A chronic disease of inflammation of the synovial lining of the joints causing pain, warmth, stiffness, redness and swelling around the joint. As this disease progresses the inflamed cells release enzymes that may digest bone and cartilage, causing loss of function and alignment, and disfiguring the shape of the joint. The cause of rheumatoid arthritis is unknown.

Scleroderma

Means 'hard skin' but it can actually affect multiple organs in the body, including the heart, lungs, blood vessels and kidneys, often causing them to shut down. Primarily affects women between the ages of 30-50 but can also strike men and children of all ages. It is a combination of an auto-immune, inflammatory and vascular disease.

Seasonal depression (seasonal affective disorder – SAD)

A depression that occurs at the same time each year, usually starting in the autumn or winter and ending in the spring or summer. Common signs are depression, sadness, anxiety, irritability, loss of interest in usual activities, fatigue, increased need for sleep, decreased energy, weight gain and increase in appetite.

Sinusitis

The sinuses are cavities in the facial bones. Lined with mucous membranes, they surround the nose and are joined to the nasal cavity. Infection, inflammation and excess mucus can block the sinuses. Severe pain can result in the forehead, upper jaw and cheekbones. Symptoms often improve after a few days but certain treatments can be used to relieve underlying infections, reduce mucus production and clear blocked sinuses.

Skin problems

Skin problems are highly visible and very common symptoms of stress. In a study conducted by Quick and Quick (1984) it was found that when eczema-prone individuals were emotionally aroused, a change in skin cells was observed.

Snoring

Occurs during sleep, usually when sleeping with an open mouth. Snoring is the noise created by the vibration of the soft palate of the mouth/throat. The noise varies from a soft sound to a loud, unpleasant noise. Can be caused by allergies, mis-positioned jaw, fat gathering in and around the throat or some other blockage in the breathing passage.

Stiffness

Lack of suppleness.

Stomach and bowel disorders

Some common stomach and bowel disorders are: ulcers, heartburn, coeliac disease, constipation, cirrhosis, diverticulitis, diverticulosis, irritable bowel syndrome, Crohn's disease. Since the stomach and bowel are key areas of digestion, it is logical that diet has a profound effect on their function.

Some people respond to stress by an increase in stomach acid which can lead to stomach ulcers. Other conditions that are thought to be brought on or aggravated by chronic stress include bleeding, ulceration and irritable bowel syndrome.

Stress

The body's reaction to stress is called the fight or flight response; a physiological mechanism designed to help a person confront difficult, fearful or dangerous situations. When the body is faced with a stressful situation it prepares to either stay and fight or take flight, by pumping out chemicals into the body.

The problem is that in the modern world, stressors are often persistent and continue to make demands on the body and mind (e.g. money worries, stress at work, relationship difficulties). This may outstrip the person's ability to deal with demands and may ultimately lead to a state of exhaustion. The symptoms of stress include: aching and tense muscles, diarrhoea, constipation, asthma, headaches, skin problems, migraines, insomnia, frequent colds, anxiety, fear, depression, anger, irritability, hostility, lack of concentration, impatience, mood swings and tearfulness.

There are many ways of dealing with stress and many of them work by initiating the relaxation response, which counteracts or decreases the stress chemicals circulating around the body, e.g. breathing and relaxation techniques, meditation and physical exercise.

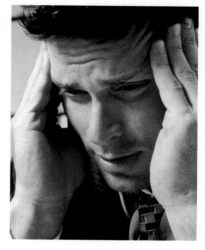

Fig. 5.13 *Work can cause stress*

Stress-related disorders

Everyday stress, when not resolved, can undermine the immune system and create a series of physical, emotional, mental and spiritual changes that can either cause illness or make existing conditions worse. Illness is often the body communicating that change of some type is required to protect your health and wellbeing.

Tension

Muscle tension is part of a vicious cycle. Even if it is not the cause of pain, it soon will contribute to it as muscle becomes tense and painful when we are worried or stressed.

Testicular disorders

The testicles produce male hormones, including testosterone, and produce sperm. Disorders affecting the testes can lead to serious complications, including hormonal imbalances, sexual dysfunction and infertility. Common problems are: trauma, due to the unprotected position of the testicles on the body; torsion, when the spermatic cord becomes twisted around the testicle, cutting off the blood supply; cancer, characterised by a lump, irregularity or enlargement of the testicle, a dull ache or pain in the scrotum, testicle, groin or lower abdomen.

Tinnitus

Tinnitus is a continuous ringing, hissing or buzzing in the ears. It can be caused by excess earwax, blocked eustachian tubes, pressure, damage or ageing. It has also been linked to the use of certain drugs such as aspirin, chloroquine and quinine, and with persistent loud noise.

Varicose veins

Enlarged, twisted, painful superficial veins caused by poorly functioning valves which impair the return of blood to the heart and allow the blood to pool.

Vitiligo

A skin disorder affecting pigmentation, causing white patches to appear on the body. Melanocytes (the cells that make pigment) in the skin, the mucous membranes, and the retina are destroyed. The cause is unknown but it is not contagious.

Wrinkles

Skin ages all over the body, but especially in areas where it is exposed to the sun, such as the face, neck and back of the hands. With age, skin cells divide more slowly and the dermal layer begins to thin. Elastin and collagen fibres, which support the outer layer, loosen and unravel causing skin to lose its elasticity. Sun exposure and smoking speed this process and cause more wrinkles to appear.

> **REMEMBER**
> Sun exposure and smoking will lead to skin wrinkling.

Progress Check

1. Give a definition of massage.
2. Which organs correlate to certain areas of the scalp?
3. How can touch help the body to heal?
4. List five effects that stress can have on the body.
5. Name five conditions where Indian Head Massage treatment has been used.

Key Terms

You need to know what these words mean. Go back through the chapter or check in the glossary to find out.

- Jiva
- Shalyakya Tantra
- Palmplan
- Stress
- Tension
- Anxiety
- Depression

Indian Head Massage for ...

After working through this chapter you will be able to:

♦ Understand the special considerations and adaptations involved in using Indian Head Massage for:

Pregnancy and childbirth
Children
The elderly
Clients with disabilities
Clients recovering from drug dependencies
Psychiatric clients
In hospitals
Care in the community
On-site Indian Head Massage (OM)
Do-it-yourself.

The basic Indian Head Massage techniques and treatments outlined can be applied to variety of clients, with different conditions and in many locations.

This chapter seeks to focus on a few of these variations and give some extra guidelines and suggestions on how to approach and adapt treatment.

Introducing Indian Head Massage in some areas of the country is relatively new. Invaluable knowledge and support is available amongst the community and so Indian Head Massage therapists should habitually give their clients additional help by making them aware that such support is available.

Equally, a responsible therapist should always work within the limits of his or her training and expertise. If a client's needs are assessed as being outside the range of the therapist's expertise, the therapist should have no hesitation in making a referral to another practitioner. Clients should be advised to consult a medical doctor about their symptoms as medical care should be seen as the primary treatment which Indian Head Massage can support.

REMEMBER
Clients should be advised to consult a medical doctor about their symptoms as medical care should be seen as the primary treatment which Indian Head Massage can support.

Indian Head Massage for pregnancy and childbirth

While pregnancy is part of the natural cycle and women's bodies are equipped and adapted to experience it successfully, pregnancy is also a period of risk for both the mother and foetus. Pregnancy also places particular demands on the emotions as well as the body of the mother.

Indian Head Massage given in pregnancy can not only help improve the mother's overall health, but can shorten the length of labour and promote a healthier outcome for mother and baby. The baby in the womb may also feel the healing effects of Indian Head Massage. During pregnancy, treatment can be general, aiming to raise the overall health of the whole body. Pregnancy is not the time to undergo any cleansing management.

REMEMBER
Indian Head Massage can help to shorten the length of labour and improve the mother's overall health.

REMEMBER
Indian Head Massage for pregnancy and childbirth should only ever by considered in consultation with the attending midwife.

You should be aware of and understand the unique features of pregnancy and bear in mind the following cautions, while always working within your range of expertise:

- If your client has a history of miscarriage, you may wish to wait until the pregnancy is well established. You should obtain advice and written consent from her doctor.
- If this is a first pregnancy or if previous pregnancy has been abnormal, offer only gentle Indian Head Massage treatments. During the first three months of pregnancy, massage may increase the risk of miscarriage.
- Common ailments that occur and relate to pregnancy include: nausea, constipation, fatigue, water retention, headaches, disturbed sleep, leg cramps, back ache, sore breast, worry and depression. As pregnancy progresses extra strains are placed on the mother's posture and circulation, which may cause problems either before or after the birth. Indian Head Massage may aid these symptoms.
- For the aforementioned reasons consideration must be given to the comfort of the client. Adjustments may need to be made in the length of the sessions as well as positioning of the client.

Receiving Indian Head Massage can relax the mother, help recovery, rebalance hormones and spinal posture and promote breastfeeding. It is normal practice in India for mother and baby to receive whole body massage for 40 days beginning three days after delivery, by therapists who specialise in pregnancy and baby massage.

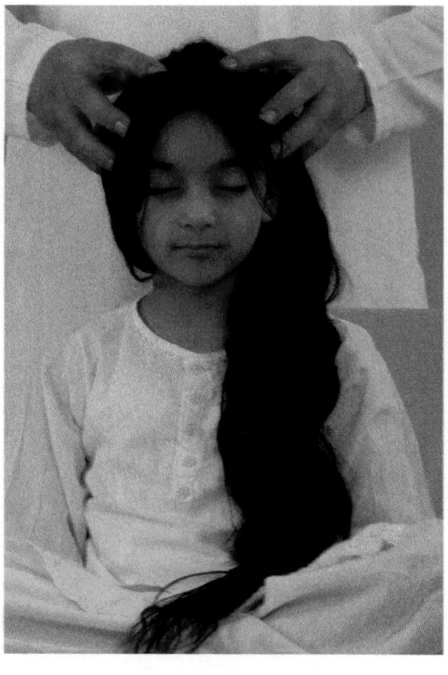

Fig. 6.01 *Treating a child with Indian Head Massage*

REMEMBER
Children are very responsive to Indian Head Massage treatment.

Indian Head Massage for children

Treating children with Indian Head Massage is both effective for the client and highly rewarding for the therapist. Children are liable to be much more responsive to treatment than adults as their minds and bodies are still relatively open and are less toxic than adults, though there are always exceptions to this. Each child must be understood as an individual. Children's inquisitive minds make them naturally open to the discovery that Indian Head Massage can have a gentle but effective influence on their health.

Benefits in treating children:

- It is a non-invasive, hence non-threatening treatment.
- Touching the head and shoulders may be acceptable whereas touching other parts of the body may be inappropriate. It can be helpful not only in physical, but also emotional, conditions.
- Teaching parents to give Indian Head Massage can facilitate bonding between parent and child and is nurturing to the child.
- It is gentle and can be a joy to do.
- It gives children a positive body image.
- Indian Head Massage may be particularly advantageous in helping children who have been abused or orphaned, or are otherwise emotionally vulnerable. It can give them the comfort and security of a loving touch, coming with unconditional concern for their welfare, helping to rebuild their self-esteem.

Indian Head Massage for the elderly

Working with the elderly can be very gratifying as this section of the population is often neglected and deprived of a nurturing touch. However, consideration must be given to the physical condition of the client prior to giving a treatment.

Bones may be brittle and joints more liable to injury. The skin may be weak and thin, circulation poor and capillaries weak, and bruising may occur easily; healing from any injury takes due care. Touch may need to be lighter. Work within the limitations of the client's range of movements, use no force and allow flexibility to increase gradually where possible.

In this group, clients may be impeded by lack of exercise, poor breathing habits and diminished capabilities of the body's systems. It has been found that for bed-ridden clients, symptoms such as anger, insomnia, fearfulness and body aches and pains, are ameliorated by Indian Head Massage.

Session length needs to be related to the condition of the client. Short but frequent sessions may be called for, especially in chronic conditions. Little but often is the key. Adjust expectations to the situation. Long-standing chronic condition may not show an obvious response for a considerable time. The treatment is still having a positive effect.

When working in nursing homes, hospitals or with clients, always obtain permission of the doctor in charge or the client's guardian before beginning treatment. It helps if you can interest the staff in Indian Head Massage. Explain the treatment and encourage them to reinforce any recommendations you make.

Find out what medication is being taken and what its effect is likely to be. Adjust your treatment accordingly. Inform the physician, nurse or family member how treatment may influence the body so that effects of medication can to be monitored and adjusted if necessary.

> **REMEMBER**
> A gentler massage may need to be given to an elderly person.

> **REMEMBER**
> Remember there are no quick fixes with Indian Head Massage treatments. Symptoms may get worse before getting better.

Indian Head Massage for people with disabilities

Indian Head Massage can be offered to people with disabilities in their wheelchair. They can therefore receive treatment in their own 'space', which can be a very welcome experience. Those with disabilities can be plagued by minor symptoms relating to their disability, which when relieved, can greatly enhance their sense of wellbeing and self-esteem. This in turn can have a knock-on effect on their relationships.

Depending on the client's disability, the following may need to be considered before giving treatment:

> **REMEMBER**
> Indian Head Massage may be given to someone in their wheelchair.

- Access to the premises and to toilet facilities
- Arrangements for the client's comfort during treatment, which may include adjustments of the wheelchair
- Arrangement for permission of parent, guardian or physician where necessary
- The handling of client's hands may need careful attention, especially if using a wheelchair.

Indian Head Massage for clients recovering from drug dependency

These clients benefit from the holistic care of Indian Head Massage just as others do. They are treated with the same respect and non-judgemental attitude. In fact the holistic approach of Indian Head Massage may enable them to better understand themselves and their condition, and to help them heal their relationship with the world, in ways that are usually not included in standard treatment.

They will learn about the nature of the prana within them, their own self-worth as an expression of that energy, how it may be hindered or helped through lifestyle, and how it may be liberated to work for them towards health through Indian Head Massage. Such knowledge fosters a positive self-image and outlook that may help them to make the necessary changes in their life.

Receiving an Indian Head Massage allows clients to experience the benefits of human touch in a safe, non-threatening environment, which may be a new experience to them. The eye contact with the therapist, re-establishment of the mind-body connections and promotion of integration over fragmentation and isolation are beneficial at all levels of being.

In western cultures, we tend to only think of drug addiction or drug abuse as the illegal use of hashish, narcotics and related substances. We do not readily acknowledge such legal forms of drug dependency as smoking, alcohol dependency, or use of prescription drugs such as Valium, amphetamines and Prozac.

Even food can be abused as if it were a drug, when it substitutes for the 'feelgood factor' or sense of self-esteem and wellbeing. We normally get these feelings from basic self-acceptance and self-love, which nurtures us and allows loving relationships with others. An eating disorder can be considered a kind of addiction, since the person is in effect using the food, or in some cases lack of it, as a means to a certain state of mind. As therapists, we should be alert to the possible incidence of such hidden dependency in our clients – often unacknowledged – as we conduct the case history. We can then advise the client or refer them to the appropriate counsellor or agency.

ACTIVITY

Put together a list of useful contact numbers for clients, such as Alcoholics Anonymous.

Whatever the drug abused, the same basic approach is taken to regain a healthy balance in the body, mind and emotions and in life habits. The therapist should also bear in mind that certain organs of the body will have been weakened by substance abuse. These particularly include the liver and kidneys. The liver works to detoxify the blood of the drug and the kidneys to balance acid and alkaline, and filter the blood of remaining impurities before excretion. If smoking is the habit, the lungs will have been congested and/or weakened. Working the eliminative areas is extremely important to cleanse the body tissues of the residue of the drugs and to nurture the energy to ease the addiction.

The client will need support through the process of recovery as there are many pitfalls awaiting them. There may be times when they feel frustrated or impatient for results or feel exhausted or depressed. They may express self-pity, blame others, or expect too much from them, or seek excuses to return to the habit.

Danger points are when some considerable progress has been made and the client feels they have mastered their weakness and need no longer abstain. They may become complacent and let up on daily disciplines, or may feel they no longer need advice and support from others, and that no one can tell them anything new. All these pitfalls and others await the client and set the stage for a relapse.

As a therapist, you should help the client to set a series of short-term realistic goals, which can be reached with normal human effort. Drug dependency has been years in the making and it will take many years of slow, steady effort to come to terms with the negative patterns that created it, and to cleanse the negative residues from the system so it can return to its natural, vibrant state of health.

Indian Head Massage should be adapted to the individual, and appropriate recommendations made during post-treatment advice. Encourage visits for further treatments on a regular basis. Indian Head Massage may not entirely bring about a complete recovery. It should be part of a multi-faceted approach involving diet, counselling, meditation and yoga, integrated with the client's present medical drug regime.

Indian Head Massage for psychiatric clients

All the benefits of balance, integration and inner communication, which are encouraged through Indian Head Massage, can greatly improve life for these clients. Here the mental and emotional aspects of treatment are to the fore; Indian Head Massage, though working primarily on the physical level, can certainly affect these.

Indian Head Massage can influence the energetic relationships between the various organs and systems and between the body and the mind. For example, healthy glandular function and healthy reproductive organs can have an effect on emotions; being full of waste in the colon can affect the head and/or heart, and cloud the understanding. A thorough cleansing on the physical level unblocks congestion, affecting the emotional and mental sphere.

Anxiety and depression can both reflect the health of the kidneys and liver, and affect these organs considerably through the stress response. Considerations about working in consultation with the client's physician and family members need to be taken into account when treating these patients; permissions may need to be obtained.

The effects of medication should be taken into account, as should the effect of Indian Head Massage treatment on the metabolism of medication. Careful monitoring of the medication dosage is needed.

Treatment sessions should be frequent and short, with the aim being for the client to have a relaxing and positive experience within the safety of the therapeutic space.

Indian Head Massage in hospitals

Many hospitals are more open to complementary and alternative medicine therapists, either in a voluntary capacity or employed as staff, than they were a few years ago. The caring therapeutic touch of Indian Head Massage gives a special welcome and support that enhances the healing processes of the mind, body and soul.

Clients welcome it because Indian Head Massage aims to treat the person, not the illness. All too often this point of view is lacking in hospitals where the focus is on controlling the disease itself. Staff receive an indirect benefit because patients will be much more comfortable and much less demanding. Indian Head Massage lends itself readily to the hospital setting.

In the hospital environment many excellent results have been achieved with Indian Head Massage in relieving clients' symptoms, including headaches, muscle aches, anxiety, weakness, irritability, feelings of insecurity and agitation. It is a very powerful tool as a non-drug approach to promoting sleep. Medical staff has found it useful for calming psychotic patients, as well as for giving rest and improving mood in depressed patients.

Indian Head Massage may be used in a variety of conditions and situations within the hospital.

- It can be used after surgery to help speed the healing of the wound and allay the shock the body has experienced.
- It is ideal as an augmentation to physiotherapy. Patients in care for psychiatric or drug dependency problems can receive benefit as described above.
- Indian Head Massage may be especially appreciated in the hospice setting.

Again the caring therapeutic touch provides much-needed comfort and helps relieve some minor symptoms of terminal illness. When working in wards within hospitals, try to ensure the maximum privacy possible. Do not aim to give a long treatment, especially in the first stages. The aim is to raise the overall health of the body by offering a very light touch.

Care in the community

A holistic approach to care recognises that our health is constantly influenced by the world around us. Indian Head Massage therapists cannot provide every aspect of care and support for a particular problem beyond our scope or knowledge. We may have a client whose health is being affected significantly by social, financial, personal or other problems which need outside help.

It is very beneficial then for the Indian Head Massage therapist to be aware of some of the major support services in the area, either local or national. There are local organisations and also local branches of national organisations, both governmental and non-governmental.

On-site Indian Head Massage (OM)

On-site massage is designed to provide maximum benefits to staff, without causing any disruption to their working day. Treatment is 20 or 30 minutes long and can be scheduled between work commitments.

Many people develop problems with their musculo-skeletal system as a result of overuse, poor posture, an inefficient working environment, lack of information or habits formed while young. These can manifest themselves as aches and pains, reduced range of motion or movement of a joint, muscle spasms, repetitive strain injury (RSI), low back pain, etc. Indian Head Massage can be used effectively in the treatment of such conditions at the client's premises.

An answer to stress

On-site massage uses an ancient Ayurvedic method called Shiro-Abhyanga. As well as rolling the muscles to release tension and reduce anxiety levels, this technique works on marma points to create a sense of balance and wellbeing. It also stimulates the blood supply, leading to increased energy. It leaves you fresh, relaxed and feeling more positive.

Immediate relief for muscle tension

These days, we spend much of our time on the telephone or at the computer. Unless we are very careful, the positions we adopt while working build up tension in muscles which can provoke stiffness or pain, and can eventually lead to serious conditions such as repetitive strain injury. Massage works directly on these muscles, relaxing them, easing stiffness and reducing tension.

Highly effective motivator

On-site massage is perceived as a valuable benefit by staff. It clearly demonstrates a strong commitment to their welfare and cultivates positive team spirit. Many companies now consider on-site massage an important part of their management philosophy.

A valuable aid to business

Stress-related illness costs businesses an estimated £20 billion a year. Massage can significantly reduce the number of working days lost, as well as providing health and wellness, an area where employers are facing increasing legal responsibilities.

Unlike other forms of stress management, the effects are immediate. Massage increases concentration and positive thinking. People return to their desks with renewed enthusiasm and vitality. They work better, not only because of the effect of the treatment, but because they have received something enjoyable and rewarding.

> **REMEMBER**
> Unlike traditional massage, with on-site Indian Head Massage no oils are used. Instead, the therapist works through the clothes, concentrating solely on the key areas of the upper body; the back, shoulders, arms, hands, neck, scalp and face.

> **REMEMBER**
> Massage can help to reduce the number of working days lost as a result of stress-related illness.

Do-it-yourself Indian Head Massage

For a do-it-yourself massage, start by taking a few deep breaths sitting in a posture that is most comfortable for you.

1. First rub your hands and then massage your temples with the fingers of each hand.
2. Next, firmly apply pressure to the scalp and forehead with all your fingers and thumbs, making small rotations, just as if you were washing your hair.
3. Very gently, rub down your forehead with your thumbs to meet your index fingers stationed on the eyebrows.
4. With your thumb and forefinger massage the earlobe all the way up to the top, pulling away from the head.
5. Finally, place your hands covering your ears, then covering your closed eyes, and finally, over the top of your head. Visualise and inhale the colour red and exhale all your worries. With each subsequent breath visualise a range of colours: red, orange, lemon, emerald, turquoise, indigo and white.

 Progress Check

1. What safety factors does the therapist need to consider prior to treating a pregnant client?
2. How can Indian Head Massage be beneficial for a pregnant client?
3. How would you modify the treatment to suit an elderly client?
4. For which conditions and situations may Indian Head Massage be used in hospitals?
5. Name three work-related conditions that can be helped by massage.

The Consultation Process and the Therapeutic Relationship

After working through this chapter you will be able to:

- Carry out a consultation for Indian Head Massage
- Understand how contraindications and precautions may affect the proposed treatment
- Liaise with other healthcare professionals
- Formulate a treatment plan for Indian Head Massage
- Know about common conditions of the head, neck and shoulders
- Know the cautions, recommendations and restrictions involved in treatment application.

Ayurveda is simply a very ancient, practical method to understand life. It begins by helping each person understand themselves and their unique nature. Then it helps one to learn how diet, lifestyle, career, family and environment interact with our nature causing balance or imbalance: health or disease; joy or sorrow. Ayurveda is a way to understand nature in precise detail. Ayurveda is an open door to health.

The human touch is one of the surest ways of unburdening stresses. Just as the embrace of a parent soothes the upset child, just as a kiss or handshake takes the sting out of an argument, the simplest touch sometimes works miracles.

Ayurveda derived in ancient societies from the spiritualistic transfer of a life force of healing power from divine healers and shamans to the sick, metamorphosing in time into the art of physical, restorative power by massage.

Ethics

As with any profession, qualified Indian Head Massage therapists have to pursue a strict code of professional ethics and conduct that must be followed at all times.

Here are a few examples of a code of ethics and professional standards for the Indian Head Massage profession:

- The therapist must never discuss clients with other clients. They must honour clients' confidentiality and privacy
- The therapist must never discuss other therapists or establishments where they work
- Only carry out treatments that are within the professional qualification; do not go against allopathic medical advice

> **REMEMBER**
> Indian Head Massage therapists follow a strict code of professional ethics and conduct.

- Conduct professional life with propriety and dignity; commit no breach of conduct or infringement of code of morality

- Respect the work of other members of the holistic and the medical health care profession
- Medical diagnosis or treatment must not be made or recommended and make no claims for results. Only make honest recommendations about treatments
- Do not treat a condition if already being treated by other therapists
- Place service before self and provide the best treatment possible, regardless of race, creed or social status

Unethical conversation

Clients come for an Indian Head Massage, like many other CAM treatments, for many different reasons. It may be they are very lonely and need someone to talk to, or their life is so hectic that they want to escape. It is part of your professional remit to be able to assess this and react accordingly.

Holistic treatments are offered in an atmosphere congenial to relaxation and an atmosphere of serenity. The client is requested to observe silence; if the client wants to chat because they are lonely, then suitable responses must be made. It is important that the conversation is 'client led'. The therapist would only issue instructions and speak when necessary – checking pressure, comfort etc. Whatever the conversation pattern turns out to be, it is vital that unethical topics are avoided. That is, anything that the client could have a strong opinion about, that the client may find upsetting, disturbing or wants to disagree with.

With experience it is possible to steer clear of these topics and keep the conversation light, conductive and professional. Examples of topics to avoid are abortion, marriage problems, money, politics, religion, sex, and any other controversial topics.

The consultation

Conducting a consultation and client consultation skills

Consultation for Indian Head Massage involves a one-to-one communication, sitting in front of the client. During a consultation, a therapist's contact with the client involves talking, listening, non-verbal communication, as well as recording written information. When carrying out a consultation, therapists need to adopt a warm, calm, open and understanding attitude towards the client, in order to facilitate a channel of positive communication.

Be kind. Everyone you meet is fighting a hard battle. Clients will come to you because they are already in a state of stress, disillusionment or lack of confidence. Having lost faith in many facets of their life, including various medicine systems, clients may come as a result of seeking an

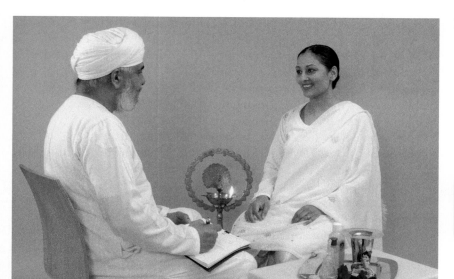

Fig. 7.01 *The consultation*

REMEMBER
Be kind. Everyone you meet is fighting a hard battle.

alternative to their present troubles. They may be apprehensive about the Indian Head Massage treatment, so it is important for a therapist to adopt a sensitive, respectful and friendly attitude towards clients at all times. An individual's quest to a more comprehensive understanding of mind, body and soul is one of the principle reasons why there is so much interest in the CAM therapies.

Imagine for a moment a bear comes and knocks on your door to say that it is in a lot of pain and bleeding because its foot got caught in a trap set by a human. Now, would you get rid of the pain the bear is in, or get rid of the trap that the bear is in?

Ayurvedic thinking employs the latter case. If you get rid of the trap that the bear is in, you get rid of the cause of the problem instead of offering it a painkiller to dispose of the pain but not the cause of the pain. Therapists need to deepen their own knowledge so that they understand as much as possible of the theory of prevention-versus-cure behind the bear trap!

REMEMBER
Always allow sufficient consultation time by asking questions regarding your client's health and past and present medical history.

A client consultation involves professional communication between a client and a therapist. Consultation is a significant skill that helps establish a positive and trusting therapeutic relationship. Build a therapeutic rapport. Always allow sufficient consultation time by asking questions regarding your client's health and past and present medical history.

Always face the client, make direct eye contact and leave no room for misunderstanding. Be precise and clear in your communication and go through the routine verbally before the hands-on treatment. A client's emotions can trigger your own emotions; looking after yourself is extremely important. Be competent and aware.

GOOD PRACTICE

Always maintain eye contact and listen carefully to the client.

REMEMBER

Apart from the delivery of a professional Indian Head Massage treatment, the therapist's second greatest ability is to be a good listener.

Apart from the delivery of a professional Indian Head Massage treatment, the therapist's second greatest ability is to be a good listener. Through effective listening and observation, a therapist can customise the treatment to meet the client's needs and expectations. It is important for therapists to realise that clients often communicate without the spoken word, and non-verbal messages may be projected without the client's awareness.

Therapists therefore need to be aware of what a client may be communicating on all levels. With this in mind, therapists may realise that there may be a difference between what a client is expressing with words and what their body language may be indicating. Occasionally 'blocks to communication' may become prevalent by the therapist. This is when you subconsciously think 'I've heard all this before'. Remind yourself that each client is different and the symptoms they have are different.

Your ability to understand the client's needs, be able to offer a treatment plan and to exercise your professional ethics, will often result in client satisfaction and their continued patronage. Therapists therefore need to have effective communication skills, which involve both talking and listening to the client, in order to be able to record and respond positively to the information elicited.

Consultation environment

REMEMBER

A calm state of mind is essential for the client to be receptive to a healing treatment. Breathing techniques can be given to centre the client and bring them to the present moment.

In order to facilitate a positive approach to a consultation, it is important to be aware of the environment in which it is undertaken. The environment for a consultation should ideally be private, in order to respect the client's privacy and dignity in disclosing personal information. Attention to aspects such as lighting, aroma, temperature and comfort of a consultation area can all help to aid client relaxation and reduce apprehension. A calm state of mind is essential for the client to be receptive to a healing treatment. Breathing techniques can be given to centre the client and bring them to the present moment.

GOOD PRACTICE

The environment during consultation should be private, clean and pleasant to be in.

Client education

Consultations provide an ideal opportunity for therapists to educate clients on what Indian Head Massage involves, its potential benefits, along with the costs and time involved. Clients do not usually want to be passive recipients of treatment. If they are to invest time and money in a therapy they need to be educated so they become partners in their healing process. Consultations also provide the client with the opportunity to ask questions about the treatment and to maintain long-term benefits.

Based on the information and the education provided about the service, the client is then responsible for making a decision as to the treatment objectives. It is the therapist's responsibility to provide a treatment to suit their needs, but to accurately inform them if their objectives and expectations are unrealistic. Also explain any reasons why it is important to encourage clients with contraindications to seek medical advice. It is essential for therapists to stress to clients the importance of regular treatments to maintain long-term benefits.

Knowledge of a client's objectives will empower therapists to make an informed decision as to a suitable treatment plan that is within safe and ethical medical guidelines. It is very important that a therapist never diagnoses a client's medical condition, and refers the client to their GP before any form of treatment is commenced.

Clients may also be empowered to take charge of their own healing through education of adjustments to lifestyle, posture and the correct use of ergonomics (Vastu – holistic concept of architecture and interior design).

Client confidentiality
Client confidentiality is an important factor in a relationship between a client and a therapist. Clients should be reassured that all information recorded will remain confidential and is stored securely, and that no information will be disclosed to a third party without the client's written consent. Maintaining client confidentiality will also help to establish a trusting professional relationship between a client and a therapist.

GOOD PRACTICE

Reassure the client that all information is confidential and stored securely.

Written documentation
Written documentation is essential in a consultation as it provides a systematic and continuing record of the client's progress. It is important to keep records and update them after every treatment. Consultation documents should always be used as a guide to facilitate communication. Questions may need to be phrased carefully to maximise communication and receive useful information. It is important for therapists to realise that information received from the client is largely subjective, in that it is from their viewpoint. This information may differ from what is evaluated by the therapist.

Focal information to be discussed during the consultation is anything which may affect the client's physical and emotional health. This includes medical history, diet, lifestyle, occupation, sleep patterns, exercise and relaxation, which will all contribute to an overall picture of the client from a holistic point of view. In addition to talking, listening and recording information on a client's records, a client consultation involves other assessment skills such as:

- Visual assessment – this commences from the first point of contact with the client. Observation as to the client's mood, rate and depth of breathing, posture and way of walking may all help to contribute to the state of the client's physical and emotional health.
- Manual assessment of the tissues – the most effective form of communication a therapist can use is touch. Throughout the Indian Head Massage treatment the therapist can assess tissues for tension, restrictions, temperature changes, etc, even though it is a clothed treatment.

It should be noted that whilst the information reflects an accurate representation of the condition in generic terms, all clients will vary in the severity of their condition. Each client should be individually assessed as to their condition at the time of the proposed treatment, and re-assessed on subsequent treatments. The guidelines given are meant as a general guide, and so therapists are encouraged to seek further clarification of a client's medical condition from the GP and from the client themselves.

Protection of client's modesty

Observe modesty/hygiene standards (personal and clinic). Provide privacy by putting a notice on doors and blinds, and curtains on windows. Give privacy for changing by providing a screen or leaving the room. Modify the massage to suit your client's body shape.

Liaising with other healthcare professionals

As the benefits of Indian Head Massage become more widely known and validated, there are more opportunities opening up for therapists to work alongside other healthcare professionals. Therapists therefore need to be aware of professional and medical etiquette when liaising with other professionals.

Referral to a healthcare professional

If a contraindication is established with a client at the time of consultation, treatment cannot usually proceed without reference to the client's GP. In this case, it is professional protocol to have a pre-prepared referral form on the therapist's stationery that the client may take to their doctor. When referring to a client's GP, it is essential that the therapist make it clear that they are seeking authorisation as to whether Indian Head Massage treatment is suitable in accordance with medical advice. In order to raise awareness of Indian Head Massage amongst healthcare professionals, it is important for therapists to include literature on Shiro-Abhyanga concerning its methodology, benefits and effects.

This is a draft layout of a letter that may be addressed to the client's doctor to obtain consent before offering an Indian Head Massage:

Date

Dear

Re: (*write client's name*) ....

Your patient, as named above, has requested an Indian Head Massage (Shiro-Abhyanga) from myself. During the consultation with the client, I understand that he/she is suffering from:

.... (*write contraindication*)

Indian Head Massage treatment increases blood circulation and helps with lymph node drainage, sinusitis, insomnia, stress, eye strain, headaches, migraine and tension in the muscles to the upper body.

I would therefore be grateful if you could indicate his/her suitability for treatment by signing the consent below.

Yours faithfully

(*Name of IHM practitioner, qualification, address and signature*)

....

Consent

I agree that the Indian Head Massage (Shiro-Abhyanga) you suggest would be suitable for this patient.

Signed ....

(*Doctor's signature, stamp and date*)

GOOD PRACTICE

Ensure that you also send a leaflet briefly explaining the treatment, as the doctor may not know what an Indian Head Massage is.

Handling referral data from other healthcare professionals

If a client has been referred to you by another healthcare professional, it is professional etiquette to reply with a status report on the client's progress. Report writing is an essential part of networking with other professionals as it helps to raise awareness of the benefits of the treatment and its value for a client's physical and emotional wellbeing. A status report should include the following information:

- A general introduction to the client and how he/she was referred
- A summary of the client's main presenting problems
- An evaluation of the therapist's findings
- The treatment used and an explanation of the techniques involved
- The client's progress
- Recommendations for future/continued treatments

Professional standards

- Give clear instructions to the client so there is no area for misunderstanding. Allow time for any questions the client may have. Ensure information to clients is clear and accurate. Issues regarding what the client can and cannot wear and where and how to sit need to be explained clearly.
- Make your clients aware of your professional qualifications for Indian Head Massage training by displaying your Professional Practitioner's Certificate.
- Conduct yourself professionally at all times even when you get to know your clients.
- Work efficiently within the professionally acceptable time for Indian Head Massage – 60 minutes. During the treatment do not cut corners or blend Indian Head Massage with other treatments.
- Adhere to a comfortable dress code (as clothes may get marked with oils wear cotton which can be washed at high temperatures) and wear clean shoes. Keep clean hair held back away from the face and wear no jewellery.
- Cover all cuts; work safely and hygienically.
- Clean, short fingernails with no varnish (clients may be allergic). Wear minimum make-up.
- Smoking should not be part of your life if you value a dedicated mind, body and spirit approach to your lifestyle. If you do smoke, brush your teeth and change into fresh clothes.

Formulating a treatment plan for Indian Head Massage

Once the verbal and non-verbal information has been elicited from the client, the therapist is then in a position to suggest a treatment plan or strategy and obtain the client's agreement before proceeding.

A treatment plan for Indian Head Massage will include the following information:

1. The date and duration of the treatment.
2. The treatment objectives and client expectations.
3. Any special considerations (such as specific areas not to be worked on).
4. Use of oils on the scalp.
5. The client's agreement.

Important information to be recorded after the treatment includes:

1. Manual and visual assessments of the client.
2. Any known reactions.
3. The result/outcome of the treatment.
4. After-care and home-care advice – use of oils.
5. Recommendations for future treatment.

Our life in the world has many difficulties without adding unnecessary self-inflicted burdens. And yet there are those who would reply that is why they took to alcohol or smoking – because of their worries. Drinking and smoking do not provide solutions. This is a life of creative work, love and hope for the future, as the atma comes in to undertake a lifetime in the light of spiritual purpose and progression.

Indian Head Massage is a very safe treatment. However, there are certain health conditions that the therapist should be aware of which may prevent treatment being carried out, or that require the client to get the permission of a doctor.

Fig. 7.03 *Consultation record*

Medical history

Name:	☐ Male ☐ Female Mr/Mrs/Miss/Other
Address:	Date of birth:
Tel no:	Marital status:
Mobile no:	Children:
Email:	Profession:

Hypersensitivity to oils? ☐ yes ☐ no	Your GP's opinion on your problems:
Hereditary profile:	
Present complaint:	Name of GP:
Current medication:	Address:
Reason for seeking treatment:	Tel:
Have you had an IHM before: ☐ yes ☐ no	Do you acknowledge a higher power in your life? ☐ yes ☐ no ☐ don't know

Have you ever suffered from any illnesses/accidents – (check contraindications)?

System	Symptom	Remarks
Cardiovascular	heart/blood pressure/thrombosis/fluid retention	
Digestive	constipation/diarrhoea/bloating/flatulence/allergies	
Endocrine	hormonal	
Integumentary	dermatitis/eczema/acne/psoriasis	
Lymphatic	cancer/cellulite/lupus	
Muscular	neck/back/legs/arms/aches and pains/rheumatism	
Nervous	epilepsy/migraine/stress/depression/tension	
Reproductive	pre-menstrual syndrome (PMS)/menopause	
Skeletal	arthritis/stiff joints	
Urinary	infection of kidney/thrush	
Immune	colds/flu/sore throats/sinuses/prone to infections	

Continued overleaf

Fig. 7.03 *(Continued)*

Lifestyle questionnaire

stress level	☐ high	☐ low	☐ average	drink water	☐ no	☐ yes	daily
energy level	☐ high	☐ low	☐ average	first intake			
hours worked			daily	eat regular meals	☐ no	☐ yes	daily
hobbies				eat vegetarian diet		%	daily
relaxation	☐ poor	☐ good	☐ average	eat between meals	☐ no	☐ yes	
exercise	☐ none	☐ regular	☐ random	last intake			
see daylight			hours	eat fruit	☐ no	☐ yes	daily
meditation/yoga	☐ no	☐ yes	☐ daily	eat vegetables	☐ no	☐ yes	daily
sleep pattern			hours	take vitamins	☐ no	☐ yes	daily
skin type	☐ oily		☐ dry	soft drinks	☐ no	☐ yes	daily
food allergies	☐ no	☐ yes		drink tea	☐ no	☐ yes	daily
Yoga	☐ no	☐ some	☐ daily	drink coffee	☐ no	☐ yes	daily
family pressures	☐ no	☐ yes		drink alcohol	☐ no	☐ yes	daily
				add salt	☐ no	☐ yes	
				add sugar	☐ no	☐ yes	
				dairy produce	☐ no	☐ yes	daily
				smoke	☐ no	☐ yes	daily

Client's declaration – I declare that the information I have given is correct to the best of my knowledge and belief. I hereby acknowledge that the nature of the treatment I am about to receive is complementary to medicine and have been fully informed about the contraindications. I am aware that my participation in this and future treatments is by my own choice.

Client signature: .... Date: ....

Contraindications

1. Conditions that are contraindicated and for which treatment cannot be provided
2. Conditions that may require referral to the client's GP or another professional before treatment may be given
3. Conditions that may present certain restrictions and for which treatment may need to be adapted
4. Special factors which may influence the treatment length or techniques applied
5. Knowledge of contraindication and precautions enables a therapist to work safely and effectively

Contraindication is a reason, symptom or situation that prevents a treatment being carried out safely. It is important that the contraindication/precautions list is checked every time a client has an Indian Head Massage treatment. Often it means missing out an area or omitting certain movements. Do not massage if either you or your client is not feeling well. <u>If in doubt, don't massage!</u>

Contraindications fall into three categories:
Totally contraindicated
- Fever/high temperature
- Acute infectious diseases
- Skin or scalp infections (herpes simplex, impetigo, ringworm, scabies, conjunctivitis, folliculitis, head lice, ringworm of the scalp)
- Recent haemorrhage
- Intoxication
- Migraine
- Recent head/neck injury

Medical advice needed
- Thrombosis/embolism
- Severe circulatory problems/heart condition
- High or low blood pressure
- Dysfunctions of the nervous system
- Epilepsy
- Diabetes
- Cancer
- Recent operations
- Osteoporosis

Localised contraindications
- Skin disorders (eczema, dermatitis, psoriasis)
- Recent scar tissue, severe bruising, open cuts, abrasions
- Undiagnosed lumps, bumps and swelling

Abdomen
During the first three months of pregnancy, massage may increase risk of miscarriage – in later pregnancy, very gentle effleurage techniques may be exercised. The abdomen should also be avoided when there is diarrhoea present.

Acne (skin problems)
You should avoid anything that looks like it should not be there, such as acne, rashes, wounds, bruises, burns, boils and blisters, for example. Usually these problems are local, so you can still massage in other areas.

AIDS
If there is no exchange of bodily fluids (blood, semen, vaginal fluids, or mother's milk), HIV (human immunodeficiency virus) cannot be transmitted during massage. However, some of the infections that people suffer from during the later stages of AIDS are contraindicated. You should avoid massaging in the case of any visible rashes, sores, lesions or swelling.

GOOD PRACTICE

If you have any cuts or scrapes or scratches on your hands, it is an especially good idea to wear thin surgical gloves while massaging an HIV-infected person with any signs of open lesions after you have approval from their doctor.

Allergies

Care should be taken to ensure that any oils or products used do not contain items to which the client may be allergic. Patch tests should be carried out to avoid adverse reactions.

Alopecia

A condition which causes either sporadic hair loss or total loss of hair across the body. This may follow illness, shock, a period of extreme stress, or may be the side effect of drug therapy (i.e. chemotherapy).

Areas of septic foci

E.g. boils, carbuncles – danger of spreading the infection.

Arthritis – Osteoarthritis

A joint disease characterised by the breakdown of articular cartilage, growth of bony spikes, swelling of the surrounding synovial membrane and stiffness and tenderness of the joint. It is also known as degenerative arthritis, is common in the elderly, and takes a progressive course affecting the weight-bearing joints – the hips, knees, and the lumbar and cervical vertebrae. This condition involves varying degrees of joint pain stiffness, limitation of movements, joint instability and deformity.

Asthma

There is considerable evidence to suggest that massage is very beneficial for asthma sufferers, especially massage around the head, neck and shoulders. Often, asthma is aggravated by stress and tension. Anything that helps to lessen tension will be of help to asthma sufferers.

> **REMEMBER**
> If the bruises or abrasions are small, you can work around them.

Bruising, open cuts or abrasions

Open wounds and abrasions in treatment areas should be avoided (massage around the area). If there is slight bleeding ensure that a plaster covers the infected area and that you do not touch it, in case of cross-infection.

Cancer

Medical clearance should always be sought before massaging a client with cancer. It is unlikely that gentle massage can cause cancer to spread through the stimulation of lymph flow, however it is important to obtain advice from the consultant medical team concerning the types of cancer and the extent of the disease. If massage is indicated, avoid massage over the area of the body receiving radiation therapy, close to tumour sites and areas of skin cancer. Light massage can be beneficial in relaxing the client and supporting the immune system.

Cardiac conditions

Always obtain medical clearance before treating a client with a severe heart condition or circulatory problem, as the increased circulation from the massage may overburden the heart and can increase the risk of angina pectoris, phlebitis, hypertension, thrombosis or embolism.

Cold sores

Cold sores are caused by the Herpes Simplex Type 1 or Type 2 viruses and can be easily spread through contact. Avoid the area of infection when doing a massage.

Cysts
Gentle movements only around the area.

Dermatitis
An inflammation of the skin, which can be caused by allergies but often the cause is unknown. Avoid the areas of inflammation.

Diabetes
Symptoms indicating diabetes include tiredness, an initial weight loss, excessive thirst, high blood pressure, hardened arteries, and altered sensations in limbs such as numbness, eyesight and urination problems, poor skin sensation and thinned skin. Massage could potentially cause tissue damage and so a doctor's consent is needed.

Dysfunction of nervous system
A light, relaxing massage may be indicated in the case of a client with cerebral palsy, multiple sclerosis, Parkinson's disease, recovering from meningitis and motor neurone disease. Massage may help to reduce spasms and involuntary movements and reduce rigidity and stiffness. Always seek medical advice before offering treatment.

Encephalitis
Means inflammation of the brain, and may cause anything from headaches to seizures. Massage may worsen the inflammation.

Epilepsy
Obtain doctor's consent first as nerves are stimulated during massage which could trigger a fit. Epilepsy is a disorder of the brain in which the patient suffers fits or convulsions. The convulsions are due to a surge of over-activity in the brain's electrical system. Some types of epilepsy may be triggered by smells; care should be taken with choice of oils or medium.

Eye infection
Conjunctivitis is when the conjunctiva of the eye becomes inflamed, red and swollen, and produces water or pus-containing discharge. Conjunctivitis may be caused by bacteria or viruses (in which case usually spreads rapidly to the other eye), or may be caused by physical or chemical irritation.

Fever/illness/high temperature
Normal body temperature changes during the day. Exercise, stress or dehydration may cause a person's temperature to go up. In these cases, it is not considered a true fever. Fever is a symptom, not a disease. A fever may mean that there is something else going on in the body that is causing it. Fever helps the body fight infections by making the body's defence systems work more efficiently. Bacteria and viruses cannot live at higher temperatures and so are killed by fever.

> **REMEMBER**
> Viral or bacterial infections circulate in the blood, therefore massage will increase the movement of infection.

Fungal infections
- Ringworm/tinea capitis, tinea barbae
  Ringworm is a fungal infection of the skin, which begins as small red papules that gradually increase in size to form a ring. Itching is pronounced with this condition and lesions may be found all over the body.

Gastro-intestinal complaints

One of the effects of gastro-intestinal conditions is dehydration, which may be aggravated by massage.

Gland disorder

- Acne
- Seborrhoea
- Rosacea

Haemorrhage

Haemorrhage is the term for excessive bleeding, which can be internal or external. Massage can cause further haemorrhaging

Head or neck injury

In the case of a recent blow to the head with concussion, or an acute neck injury such as whiplash, it would be inadvisable to treat due to the risk of exacerbating the condition and increasing the inflammation and pain. However, if there is an old injury, massage may help to reduce scar tissue, decrease pain and increase mobility. Always obtain medical clearance to ensure the client's condition is suitable for treatment. If the injury is minor, such as a pulled muscle in the neck or shoulders, gentle massage will benefit the client.

Hepatitis

Avoid open lesions on the client and yourself, and wash all surfaces (chair, table, linens, towels, clothing, hands etc.). Hepatitis, like HIV, is most effectively transferred through blood and sexual fluids.

High/low blood pressure

Only with doctor's consent. Movements can increase pressure, which could result in a stroke.

Low blood pressure (hypotension) is when the blood pressure is below normal for a substantial time. Blood pressure must therefore be sufficient to pump blood to the brain when the body is in the upright position. If it is not then the person might feel faint.

Therapists are advised to carefully monitor a client's reaction and advise clients to get up slowly after treatment. Massage is usually found to be soothing and relaxing.

Hypertrophic disorders

- Basal cell carcinoma
- Squamous cell carcinoma
- Malignant melanoma

Influenza (flu)

Flu is a contagious respiratory illness caused by the influenza viruses. It can cause mild to severe illness, and at times can lead to death.

> **REMEMBER**
> Vigorous exercise can cause minor tearing of muscle fibres and is thought to be a major reason why muscles become sore and stiff 12–28 hours afterwards.

Symptoms of flu include:

- Fever (usually high)
- Headache
- Extreme tiredness
- Dry cough
- Sore throat
- Runny or stuffy nose
- Muscle aches
- Stomach symptoms, such as nausea, vomiting, and diarrhoea, can also occur but are more common in children than adults

Viral or bacterial infections circulate in the blood therefore massage will increase the movement of infection.

Infestations

- Parasitical lice, pediculosis and scabies
  Lice are tiny, white insects that may live on skin or hair. Scabies are tiny mites that burrow under the skin and lay eggs and are often found between folds of skin on the fingers and toes, wrists, underarms and groin. Both cause intense itching. Do not massage a client with either of these infections.

> **REMEMBER**
> Cross-infection could occur if you carry out a massage on someone with an infestation of lice.

Inflammatory skin disorders

- Contact dermatitis
- Eczema
- Psoriasis
- Seborrhoeic dermatitis
- Hives
- Dandruff/pityriasis simplex capitis

Inflammation and pain

For example, rheumatoid arthritis, gout, thrombosis or embolism, phlebitis, acute sprain, gastro-enteritis or any condition where the skin is swollen, red, hot and painful to touch. Never treat as a clot can be dislodged and circulate to vital organs.

Intoxication

Recreational drugs or alcohol increase blood flow to the head which could make the client feel dizzy and nauseous.

Lumps, bumps and swelling

The client should be referred to their GP for a diagnosis. Massage may increase the vulnerability to damage in the area by virtue of pressure and movement.

Medication

Indian Head Massage treatments may be of benefit as part of an allopathic health programme, where it has the potential to stimulate the body to heal itself and to reduce the rate of progress of the prevailing medical condition. Indian Head Massage's holistic approach may be used as part of the client's relaxation routine and may well have the potential to combat the side effects of certain necessary drug regimes.

Certain medications may inhibit or distort the client's ability to give feedback regarding pressure, discomfort and pain.

GOOD PRACTICE

Always check with the client's GP if you are unsure as to the type of medication and its effects.

Metal plates

Use caution when massaging a client who has a metal plate inserted in his or her body. Gentle massage may be very beneficial in the case of plates located around joints as it calms muscle tension and spasms.

REMEMBER
Indian Head Massage treatment can help to prevent the onset of headaches or migraine.

Migraine

Never treat anyone with a migraine attack. For a 'normal' headache it is safe to treat with gentle movements.

Psychotic conditions

Most psychotic conditions fall into these groups:

- Thought or perceptual disorders (e.g. schizophrenia)
- Mood disorders with psychosis (bipolar disorder)
- Psychotic disorders due to other diseases or conditions (Alzheimer's disease).

While many of these conditions will benefit from massage, it is prudent to have the client get approval from their doctor before treating.

Pyrexia

This is defined as the presence of a fever of 38°C or more, in the first 14 days after a woman has given birth. There are many causes of such a fever, but in the days prior to antibiotics it had a very poor prognosis. These days, with prompt recognition and treatment of the underlying cause, the outcome is considerably better.

REMEMBER
Gentle massage may be applied over healed scar tissue in order to help break down adhesions.

Recent scar tissue

Massage should only be applied once the tissue is fully healed and can withstand pressure.

Recent surgery

Depending on the site of the surgery, it may be necessary to obtain medical clearance before carrying out treatment.

Rheumatoid arthritis/osteoporosis/spondylitis/spondylosis

Due to brittleness of bones and possible fusion, movements should be carried out with care.

Scalp infections

It is important for therapists to avoid all contact with lesions. A client with any skin or scalp infection should be advised to seek advice and treatment from their GP.

- Folliculitis is a bacterial infection of the hair follicles of the skin and appears as a small pustule at the base of a hair follicle. There is redness, swelling and pain around the hair follicle.
- Pediculosis (lice) is an infestation (wingless insect) that feeds on human and animal blood. With head lice, nits may be found in hair. Nits are pearl-grey or brown oval structures found on the hair shaft close to the scalp. The scalp may appear red and raw due to scratching. A client affected by body lice will complain of itching especially in the shoulder, back and buttock area.
- Tinea capitis is a fungal infection of the scalp (ringworm) and appears as painless, round, hairless patches on the scalp. Itching may be present and the lesion may appear red and scaly.

Skin conditions
- Bacterial infections
- Boils
- Conjunctivitis
- Folliculitis
- Impetigo – a superficial contagious inflammatory disease caused by streptococcal and staphylococcal bacteria. It is commonly seen on the face around the ears, and features include weeping blisters, which dry to form honey-coloured crusts
- Stye

Skin infections
Never treat any contagious or infectious skin conditions or diseases as they may be worsened and spread by the massage.

Thrombosis/embolism
There is a theoretical risk that a blood clot may become detached from its site of formation and be carried in the body to another part. Always refer to the client's GP for advice on the severity of the condition before offering treatment.

Undiagnosed acute pain
If the pain is muscular, massage will help to relax the area. If there is any question regarding the origin of the pain, ask for a doctor's approval.

Untreated severe medical conditions
These clients should not be massaged without a doctor's written consent.

Varicose veins
Increased risk of bursting, and can be painful.

Viral infections
- Herpes simplex/cold sores – the condition is normally found on the face and around the lips. It begins as an itching sensation, followed by erythema and a group of small blisters, which then weep and form crusts. The condition normally persists for approximately two to three weeks but will reappear at times of stress, ill health or exposure to sunlight.

- Shingles/ herpes zoster
- Warts are caused by the human papilloma virus. They are highly contagious and should be considered a localised contraindication for massage – avoid contact. If the wart is located on the hands of the therapist, make sure the area is well covered by a plaster.

Contra-actions

At the start of a series of Indian Head Massage treatments, short-term responses may occur in the form of symptoms. These responses may become apparent in terms of:

Table 7.01

Symptom	Reason
Tiredness	Due to release of toxins which flood the system and also to the initiation of healing energies which require the body to rest in order to help to heal
Aching and soreness within muscles	The tiredness experienced after massage is usually replaced by invigorated and refreshed feeling after the treatment
Heightened emotional state	Due to release of toxins and the nerve fibres responding to the deep work undertaken
Occasionally Headache Dizziness or nausea Disrupted sleeping pattern Increased release of mucus in the ENT area	Cleansing of the mind and emotions due to re-balancing of the chakras These reactions are normal and show that toxins are being released

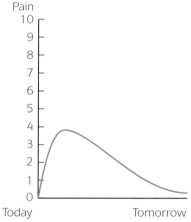

Pain

Fig. 7.04 *The long-term benefit of IHM*

These responses will ease off in no time. They show that the body is still capable of developing self-regulation and reveal that the healing process is in progress. Always remember that complementary medicine will address the root cause of the disease and some clients' symptoms might get worse before getting positively better. A little time each day spent on your health may prevent a long time spent with illness in the future.

Progress Check

1. Why must a therapist follow a code of ethics?
2. State three reasons why consultations are important.
3. What would you do if a client informed you they suffered with high blood pressure?
4. List ten contraindications to Indian head massage.
5. Why is it important to formulate a treatment plan for your client?

Key Terms

You need to know what these words mean. Go back through the chapter or check in the glossary to find out.

- Ethics
- Consultation
- Treatment plan
- Contra-actions
- Contraindications

After working through this chapter you will be able to:

◆ Learn how to create the right ambiance for the treatment room, the client and the therapist
◆ Identify the right methods of hygiene
◆ Learn about employment standards.

A healing space

In every town and city there are clinics – hundreds and thousands of them all over the country, and your clinic is one of them. It might be in a house or in a room in a commercial building. Whatever your personal/financial circumstances your practice could be a special experience for anyone who comes to visit you, leaving noise, gossip, bright lights, graffiti, sadness, bickering and perhaps worry outside.

GOOD PRACTICE

Remember it is important that the client feels relaxed in the treatment room and that you create the right ambience.

To heal is to make better. Does your clinic make clients feel better for having been in it? Do they go away feeling warmed and strengthened by the oasis you have created? Imagine a place where you could go after a day of hospital visiting or looking after toddlers, or dealing with the deadlines and personalities at work. When you walk through the door, how would it be?

In a healing space you would sense peace and quiet, welcome, a smile, space, stillness and serenity. You would not be met by newspapers, television commercials or heavy music. The pictures on the walls take your eyes up winding paths through fields, or take you to stand by the sea and watch the waves; in a vase there are simple flowers or even a spray of leaves. It would be light and airy, the coolness would flow over you. Or it could be cosy with the warmth of welcome, a place to curl up in.

Heal someone who might be wounded in their soul. Do you allow clients to be themselves providing the space and the kindness where they can share their concerns and not feel in competition with your difficulties? Healing happens when we tune in to what is beyond the surface. To come to a healing space is to receive encouragement and a listening ear, to hear some good news, to feel a smile coming back. It is a place where, for a short time away from the outside world, shoulders can drop down, breathing and pulse rate slow down, and stomachs stop churning.

Many clients need an oasis – not just friends and family. Could you make your clinic a healing space? With a little gift for clients to take away with them – perhaps one or two flowers or vegetables, or a card with a message of hope, perhaps a surprise package – the healing will continue long after the visit. The memories of the visit will say 'that was nice!' A happy mind is medicine; no better prescription exists.

What about you? When you have given cheer, expecting nothing in return, you will find that you have been refreshed. You will feel tired maybe, but warmer. Your own problems are still there, but you are stronger to bear them. Mentally wrap them up and put them out. They do not belong to either of you now, for healing has begun. We make a living by what we get, we make a life by what we give.

Your work environment reflects your personality. How you set up your practice room affects the client and their trust in you. You must choose a personal style that is comfortable for you and keep your space clean and hygienic. You should look, act and be professional, yet relaxed. Your oils and towels should be well kept, professional-looking and easy to use. Incense, flowers, plants and music are all useful to make a good environment for Indian Head Massage.

GOOD PRACTICE

Remember the practice room should always be clean, tidy and hygienic.

Ambience

The treatment room should be warm and comfortable and a safe environment. It should be clean, clear of clutter, private, quiet, well ventilated and draught free, with subdued lighting. The fragrance of burning incense and music playing softly in the background encourages relaxation.

Fig. 8.01 *A treatment room*

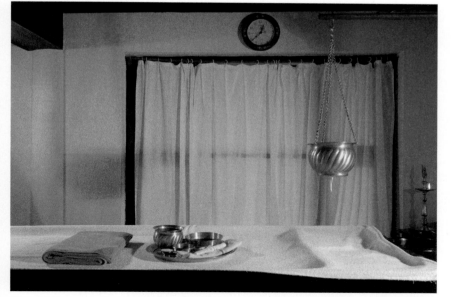

Use light colours to co-ordinate the room and wooden floors or tight woven carpet in a neutral colour (beige, brown or light green) for opulence. When designing the practice room and the environment, consider the use of natural fibres – wood and cotton can create an earthy, relaxing feeling.

Disconnect the telephone in the practice room and ask your family and friends not to enter the room. In fact, install a sign outside the door displaying 'do not disturb'.

Breathing

Every cell of our bodies needs air. We need to exchange the carbon dioxide in our lungs for fresh oxygen. How does this happen? We breathe. Even as you have been reading these few lines, your chest has been rising and falling, and you may not have even thought about it.

An adult breathes about 16 times a minute. In a day that amounts to about 2,000 litres of air, that travels at 50 km an hour as we breathe in and out. Coughs or sneezes can reach 750 km an hour! When we breathe we use our lungs, which are like sponges with 300 million little pockets providing an immense surface area, which is where the gases are exchanged.

Every cell in our bodies needs oxygen to function well. Many of us do not get the full amount of oxygen we need. This can be for a variety of reasons.

- Exercise – if we do not exercise and get out of breath regularly then our lungs become weak.
- Insulation – our homes, office blocks and other public buildings are often insulated to keep in the heat and save energy. Some have almost sealed systems. As a result we rarely breathe any new air. This leads to an increased risk of moulds, bacteria, house mites and other disease-laden organisms which thrive in these conditions.
- Overeating – if the stomach is very full, there is less room for the lungs to expand to their full extent.
- Overweight – if we have fat around our body there is constriction of the cavity around our lungs.
- Pollution – fumes, particles in the air, gases from manufactured goods, and second-hand cigarette smoke all decrease the amount of oxygen we can take into our lungs. If we took an air sample of 1 cubic inch (16 cubic cm) of air mid-way across the Pacific Ocean it would have only 15,000 particles in it. If we took a similar sample in a city it could have 5 million particles. Most people live in cities!
- Posture – if we sit up, or stand or walk with a straight back, our lungs can work more deeply and we can breathe better.
- Shallow breathing – for many reasons, including stress or sitting too much, many people only breathe with the top half of their lungs. This shallow kind of breathing that does not open up the bottom of the lungs regularly leads to infections and other respiratory problems.
- Smoking – small moving parts, called cilia, are paralysed by cigarette smoke and cannot do their job of cleaning the air the smoker breathes. With each puff of a cigarette the passages in the lungs narrow making it hard to get oxygen into the blood to go round the body. Black tar also accumulates in the tissues.

REMEMBER
A poor posture can lead to aches and pain and can restrict breathing.

- Tight clothes – any garment that is tight around our chest or waist restricts our lungs and affects how much oxygen we get.

Are there any of these that you need to correct to make full breathing easier for you? The more oxygen you can have in your body the better you will function, and the better health you will have. Prana also comes with breath.

Today we live in centrally heated homes, travel in vehicles with recycled air (to avoid pollution while keeping warm), and fly in planes with sealed oxygen systems, breathing each other's germs for hours at a time. We work in office blocks and buildings that are sealed so that windows are never able to be opened, visit or stay in hospitals or residential homes where people rarely see the outside world, and we spend time in pubs, restaurants, clubs, theatres, cinemas or supermarket complexes.

Some of these have no windows, some are heavy with cigarette smoke, and others have all man-made fabrics or recycled air. In the course of a normal day many of us hardly ever breathe negatively-ionised, real, fresh air that has blown over oceans, fields and forests.

When we breathe we take in oxygen, but our bodies only hold onto a fifth of it, and the rest is exhaled. What if the air we breathe to start with has a very low amount of oxygen? We need oxygen for making new cells, fighting disease and for thinking. How many times a day do you breathe air outside a building?

Music

Music can play an effective role in helping us lead better, more fruitful lives. Listening to specific kinds of music at specific times of the day has been shown to be helpful in maintaining good health. Classical Indian music with its many Ragas (scales) is known to be particularly therapeutic.

> **REMEMBER**
> Music can help a client to relax during treatment.

Naad Brama is the sister volume to Ayurveda. The ancient musicologists were particularly interested in the effect of music and how it affected and enhanced human behaviour. Music has potency from cure to mood swings. Extensive research suggests that the effects of each Raga (male) or Ragini (female) have an association with a definite mood or sentiment, that nature arouses in the human being.

One of the unique characteristics of Indian classical music is the assignment of definite times of the day and night for performing certain Raga/Ragini, which reflect their melodic beauty and majestic splendour.

There are some Ragas which are very attractive in the early hours of the mornings, others which appeal in the evening, and others which spread their fragrance only near the midnight hour.

This connection of time with the Raga or Raginis is based on the daily cycle of changes that occur in our own body and mind. Different moments of the day arouse and stimulate different moods and emotions.

The curative power of music emanates from the resonance of certain Ragas/Raginis on hormonal and glandular function, which produces secretions that keep the body balanced and infection free. It is believed that music stimulates the pituitary gland whose secretions affect the nervous system and the flow of blood.

For example, the Raga Kedar aids the relief of headaches, the common cold, coughs and asthma.

Furnishings
Two chairs
In your treatment room you will need one chair for yourself while interviewing the client, and one low-backed chair for the client during treatment.

Coat rack/coat hangers
Hang up your client's coat to keep your work area tidy.

Cupboard
Use a chest of drawers to store materials away dust-free.

Curtains/blinds
Window coverings provide privacy and allow you to control the lighting in your work area.

First-aid box
Make sure the supplies in your first-aid kit are kept current. Replace items when used and store in an easily accessed location. If kept inside a cupboard or drawer, mark on the outside where it is located. The kit should include plasters, bandages, wound dressings, safety pins, eyepads and cleaning wipes.

Green plants or fresh flowers
Fresh plants or flowers add a natural element to the ambience of your treatment area.

Laundry basket
Use to hold towels and any other linen until it can be laundered.

Qualification – Indian Head Massage certificate
After training, when you receive your certificate, mount it in a suitable frame and display it proudly in your working area.

Trolley/tray
Use to keep oil, hair clips, towels and any other necessary supplies close at hand.

Waste paper bin with lid
Collect refuse in a bin with a lid. Empty frequently.

Client care
Blanket/large towels
Use a blanket or large towel to wrap the client's body or to place over them if needed for warmth. Use clean, thick, soft towels that have been pre-warmed on a radiator if cold. Use one medium-size towel to go around the client's neck and another to cover the scalp after treatment.

Box of tissues
Have tissues available if needed by the client.

Carrier oil
Sesame oil is used to enhance effectiveness of treatment.

Comb
Keep a comb close by, in case it is needed by the client following treatment. Clean after each use.

Footstool/cushions
Cushions can be used to improve your client's comfort during treatment. If a footstool is not available, use a cushion for resting their feet.

Hair clip
To hold back long hair.

Oil container
Do not use oil directly from its original bottle. Lightly warm the oil over a candle burner. A smaller, flip-top plastic bottle will allow for easier application during treatment. Refill as required.

Plate for body adornments
Have clients remove their jewellery and place it on a plate under their chair, or in a place where they can keep it in sight. Remind clients to retrieve it after their treatment.

Water bottle and glass
Offer your client a drink of water at the end of your session and encourage them to increase their water intake following treatment.

GOOD PRACTICE

Offer your client a glass of water at the end of the treatment.

Therapist care and employment standards

As a therapist you must be aware of yourself or your clients will be affected by your state of mind. The more refined your mind, the better work you will be able to do and the broader base of clientele you will be able to treat.

You cannot give what you don't have. 'A woman brought her child to Mahatma Gandhi and asked him to tell her child to stop eating sugar. Gandhi told her to come back after a week. When the two returned, Gandhi told the child to stop eating sugar. The mother looked on and asked, "Why didn't you tell my son last week instead of asking us to come back?" Gandhi replied, "Last week I was still eating sugar."'

Professional life
- A client's emotions can trigger your own; looking after yourself is extremely important; be competent and aware
- Conduct professional life with propriety and dignity; commit no breach of conduct and infringe no code of morality

Professional appearance

Fig. 8.02 *The therapist's appearance is very important*

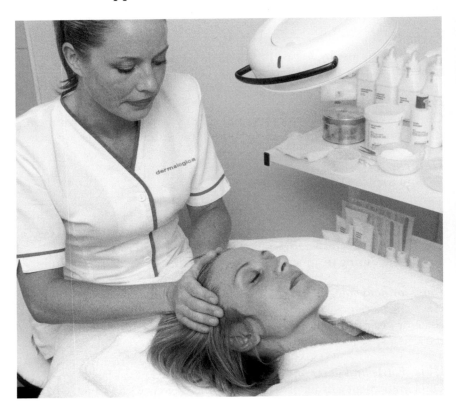

When you are clean, well groomed and attentive to caring for yourself and your appearance, you reassure your clients that you take care in all that you do. First impressions count. The therapist must always look clean and neatly presented.

GOOD PRACTICE

A professional therapist should be clean, well groomed and wear appropriate clothing.

Before conducting any treatment, the therapist should have trimmed nails, removed any jewellery and have freshly washed hands. Wear appropriate professional clothing. It not only enhances the professionalism of the therapist but also protects the therapist's clothing from the oil.

You need to consider the following when offering Indian Head Massage treatments:

- Clean short nails with no varnish
- Minimum make-up
- Clean hair held back away from the face
- No jewellery
- Cover all cuts to work safely and hygienically
- Comfortable dress code with clean shoes
- Shake your hands, arms and body to loosen up
- Exercise a regular hand-massage routine
- If you smoke, brush your teeth and change into fresh clothes

Posture

The position in which the body is held while working depends on:

- Flexibility of the joints
- Training to improve muscle power
- State of health, weight and physical fitness
- Mood – whether happy, depressed, tired, angry, etc.

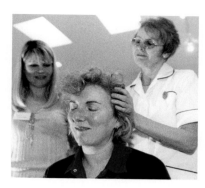

Fig. 8.03 *Good posture*

Good standing posture, when the spine is kept in its natural shape, occurs when:

- The head is held up.
- The shoulders are held back in a relaxed manner.
- The lower part of the back is hollow.
- The abdominal muscles are held in firmly and give support to the lumbar region of the backbone.
- The weight is well balanced on the feet. Any adjustment in height should be exercised by distribution of weight through the legs.

Ethics and behaviour

Cultivate a reputation of integrity by treating your clients the way you would like to be treated. Attention to ethics should be part of your everyday life. Demonstrate that you recognise and value each individual's inherent worth as you share your time, knowledge and expertise with your clients, your co-workers and your friends and family.

- Behave professionally, treat family and friends the same as clients.
- Minimise waste of oils.
- Present clear instructions.
- Allow time for any questions from the client.
- Work efficiently within the professionally acceptable time of 60 minutes, from consultation to post-treatment advice.
- The guiding principles for Shiro-Abhyanga are:
  Go slowly
  Be gentle
  Keep within the client's comfort zone.

> **REMEMBER**
> Poor posture puts the muscles out of balance. If it becomes a regular habit, those muscles and ligaments which are put under extra strain will tire more easily and begin to ache.

Protection
Sage

Before Christianity arrived in the West, the herb sage was burnt to consecrate a ritual space and was carried as a herb of protection. Sage absorbs negativity and misfortune. It drives away disturbances and tensions, and lifts the spirits above the mundane cares of life. In many parts of the Americas and Europe, it is still a very important tool with traditional healers.

Sacrament uses:

- Western tradition holds that those who eat sage become immortal in wisdom and in years.
- It claims to bring wisdom, immortality, wealth, esteem, long life and good health.
- It is used to attract money.
- English herbalists believed that in the garden this plant would prosper or wane as the owner's business prospered or failed.
- In France, it was displayed in cemeteries to mitigate grief.

> **REMEMBER**
> Sage absorbs negativity and misfortune.

- It was also said that the plant grows vigorously in any garden where the wife rules the house. As a result, it was common for the husband to prune the garden ruthlessly to destroy the evidence of his subservience.

Domestic virtues:
- Use in prosperity charms to draw money.
- Add to incenses intended to bring on restful states for meditation.
- If induces sleep if burned.
- Sprinkle it around the house to ward off hexes.

So in effect when you burn an incense stick, you are sanctifying your treatment space. During Ayurvedic treatments, a therapist performs this rite by burning the aromatic incense sticks also known as dhoof and agarbati. Burning sage achieves the same effects.

Prayer
Prayer is communication with a Source/God/Goddess in any language, where all prayers are heard.

'Not wounded by weapons, not burned by fire, not dried by the wind, not wetted by water, such is the Atma (Soul).' *Vedas.*

Almost all major modern religions, except Hinduism, are about 2000 years old. Ayurveda, Tantra and Yoga have enjoyed an immortal life and teach that we are first beings of energy, then human beings. The above quotation describes the soul as being indestructible, which can only equate to the Source.

Ayurveda is energy (prana) medicine. Our bodies are churches/temples for the Source of energy to dwell in. We have a very important task to look after our bodies, as they are the host to life. Communicating with the Source in your home or clinic can be performed in many ways from a thought to singing. Always ask for protection over your treatment engagements, then encapsulate your aura in a golden-white light.

As we connect with clients on a physical level, we also connect on a spiritual and psychic level. Take time to centre and protect yourself to avoid psychic 'burn-out'. Before each session take time to prepare yourself, your treatment space and pre-treatment meditation. Draw and transmit energy from your breath rather than using your muscle power which may tire you.

Psychic protection
Psychic defence for both the therapist and client is mandatory. Its purpose is to protect the therapist from becoming host to the client's negativity and vice versa. Energies communicate at a level beyond our understanding.

In a certain situation, a person may perceive you in a particular way while you might get the feeling that you don't want to go there again. People normally associate this type of situation with negative energy. The Source, however, does not create positive or negative energy, negative or positive vibrations may have an implication on the subject matter. Sometimes after delivering or receiving a treatment the client or therapist may feel weak and drained of their personal energy levels.

Regular pranayama coupled with meditation will aid your concentration and will sanctify your mind and body so that your pranic stock may be enhanced. The earlier in the morning that you can make an effort to sit and meditate the better opportunity you have to attract potent prana.

Environmental protection

A diva is an Indian light lamp – a miniature clay pot containing ghee with a cotton wick that, when lit in temples and auspicious occasions in the home, is considered to consecrate and purify the location.

Pure beeswax is one of nature's most perfect products. Prized since ancient times, fragrant beeswax candles burn longer and cleaner than ordinary wax candles. In fact, pure beeswax has the highest melting point of any known wax. Its slow, smokeless flame gives off more light and heat than other waxes and there's no dripping. Made by industrious honeybees from the nectar of flowers, beeswax has a sweet, natural fragrance all its own. Don't be fooled by 'aromatherapy' candles which may contain synthetic substances which could cause irritation to the client.

Beeswax is the only fuel known to science that releases a negative ion as it burns. Negative ions are proven to eliminate dust, pollen, mould, smoke and food odour as well as airborne germs and bacteria. These ions are nature's way of cleaning up man's pollution. They are a fundamental aspect of our planet's survival and are found in high concentrations in several ecological areas like mountain regions, seashores, waterfalls and oceans. Electrical storms and rainfall also release a tremendous number of negative ions. They help alleviate asthma and allergies and invigorate the most basic cells of the human body.

Beeswax burns with a brilliant, golden flame that will enhance any spiritual experience. Its positive vibrations will charm and illuminate – bringing heightened connection, awareness and constructive energy to any gathering or meditative session. Bees will travel over 50,000 miles and pollinate over two million flowers to generate 100g of pure beeswax. Beeswax is actually white, but turns yellow due to the natural colour of pollen. The sweet aroma is the true essence of 10,000 flowers. It comes in a variety of shades and tones depending on the region and the nectar's source from which it is harvested. It is interesting to note that the various shades of beeswax and honey resemble the skin tones of every human being on earth.

Beeswax was traditionally used in art, religious ceremonies, as a cloth preserver and in healing ointments. Today it is used in candles, cosmetics, salves, waterproofing, tool maintenance, furniture preserving, carpentry and in the grafting of plants and trees. Because of its purity and natural origins, beeswax burns on the identical light spectrum as fire: a source that is conducive to the relaxation of the retina (of the eye) and thus helps

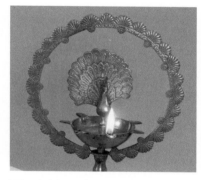

Fig. 8.04 *A diva – necessary to protect yourself from a client's negative vibrations, and, more importantly, to replenish your own stock of Prana*

to ease tension in the body's central nervous system. These candles produce a very bright flame and are ideal for meditation, relaxation and yoga. The connection between the bee and a 'higher power' can be traced back to ancient times. It is customary that candles burned in churches be made from beeswax: the significance being that the bee literally processes the nectars of the Gods.

Oils

Any substance that is put on the skin is absorbed immediately into the plasma and then into the blood and muscles. Hence, chemicals or other inorganic substances that are applied to the skin are carried throughout the body by the blood and plasma. They are not confined to the skin alone. When these substances enter into the body there is disturbance of the metabolism, minor or major depending on the substance and frequency of application. The long-term effect of any inorganic substance is to suppress or restrict the metabolic process in the body. This forms toxic material, or ama, in the body. Ama is generally described as undigested food matter in Ayurveda. Nonetheless, ama is of a mental nature, as well as a physical nature. Other physical forms of ama (toxins) are created by the substances we put on our skin.

Why are oils so good for the body? Because they are food. In classical Ayurveda all forms of oily products, from butter and ghee to vegetable fats, were used and classified according to their therapeutic actions.

Vegetable oils contain many vitamins, minerals, enzymes and prana that strengthen and nourish the body. However, to actually get these qualities from the oil, the oil itself must be 'cold pressed'. This means that the extraction process of getting the oil from the seeds or vegetable, etc., must be done without heat or chemicals.

The use of oil is important in the prevention and elimination of toxic waste in the body. Massage therapy with quality oils increases the agni (digestive fire) in the body.

The use of virgin vegetable oils in the massage of the scalp can have a strong influence on the quality of your hair care. Hair growth is stimulated as regular Indian Head Massage with vegetable oils keeps the hair strong and lustrous. Massaging the scalp stimulates the flow of blood to the follicles, thus bringing the nutrients necessary for a healthy head of hair. The secret of strengthening hair and scalp is to oil hair with virgin oils that harmonise one's dosha.

When oil is applied to the head, it gets absorbed deep into the scalp through the roots of the hair. This nourishes, lubricates and strengthens the hair roots and the skin of the scalp, preventing hair loss and premature greying. It improves circulation to the head, relaxing the muscles and nerve fibres. This helps to refresh both the mind and the body, relieving tension and fatigue and improving the complexion.

Massaging the head will increase the flow of fresh oxygen and glucose to the brain and improves the circulation of the spinal fluid around the brain and spinal cord. It also increases the release of hormones and enzymes necessary for the growth of the brain and relaxation of the body. As massage to the head increases the prana, the use of oil should be mandatory in a traditional approach. Western women may find it difficult to accept the idea of oil in their hair and scalp, but it is worth considering investment in inner beauty.

'One who regularly applies oil on the head does not suffer from headaches, baldness or premature greying hair, and generates profound sleep and peace. The hair retains its lustre and the skin of the face is rejuvenated. Massage of the head will strengthen scalp, forehead, and enlighten the senses.' *Ayurveda texts*

The skin is the body's largest organ. It absorbs up to 70% of whatever is put onto it, directly into the body and so it is important to choose organic massage oils. Inorganic oils, lotions, creams and mineral oils all clog the systems of the body, suppressing immune function and increasing toxic waste. It is good to remember, 'Never put on your body what you wouldn't eat'.

Indian Head Massage is particularly beneficial before bathing in the morning, to gently awaken the nerves. In the evening it helps remove the stress of the day and promotes peaceful sleep. Oiling the feet is also very helpful for deep, refreshing sleep as it tames Vata and banishes worries.

> **REMEMBER**
> Using oils while giving Indian Head Massage treatment will help to keep the hair strong and lustrous.

Hands cannot apply pressure while moving smoothly over the surface of the skin without some kind of lubricating agent. Oil fulfils this function better than anything else does. Two kinds of oil most commonly used for massage are vegetable and mineral. In the West, mineral oil is used in most professional clinics and spas because it is cheaper. Organic vegetable-based oils are easily absorbed and add vitamins to the skin.

Never blend essential oils/herbs/spices with virgin base oils for Indian Head Massage treatment, as they will quickly escape into the bloodstream and may have a sedative effect on the client. The client should be advised to leave the oil on the scalp and hair as long as possible after the treatment, preferably overnight. Always check if the client is hypersensitive to oils or suffers from a nut allergy before using oil during the treatment.

Benefits of scalp oil massage
- Stimulates blood circulation which nourishes the scalp and improves the scalp condition
- Builds and maintains strong muscles, nerves and connective tissues
- Loosens scalp muscles to relieve tension
- The oil will condition and moisturise dry hair and scalp
- Nourishes the skin and muscles
- Cleanses and enriches the blood

Benefits and effects of use of oil
- Helps relieve muscular aches, pains and stiffness
- May prevent hair from turning grey
- Moisturises dry skin and hair
- Improves the skin's resilience
- Warms the body

Massage with oils in Ayurveda nourishes the mind and body creating a deep inner balance. For this reason, much importance is given to spreading oil evenly over the skin so that it can be properly absorbed.

Sesame oil is found to be best for most clients, because it settles all the three dosha types and nourishes the body. If sesame does not agree with your client (e.g. if it causes acne or they are allergic to it), you may use olive oil in the cooler months and coconut during summer.

Sesame oil is a thick liquid with a golden/yellow colour and a slightly nutty aroma. It is extracted from sesame seeds and is the most popular oil used in India, especially in the summer months. Sesame seeds are rich in vitamin E and minerals such as iron, calcium and phosphorus, which help nourish and protect the hair and skin.

Research in the last 30 years has confirmed that the skin can indeed ingest oily substances. Sesame oil contains unusually large amounts of linoleic acid (compared to coconut, olive and other vegetable oils). The quality and effectiveness of a treatment rests largely in the quality and characteristics of the oil used.

Sesame oil has a unique value even from the perspective of modern science, since its chemical structure gives it a unique ability to penetrate most surfaces. This is an important element of the oil massage. The ancient Ayurvedic texts make it clear that much of the benefit derives from oil being absorbed through the skin.

REMEMBER
Sesame oil is best for most clients, because it settles all the three doshas types and nourishes the body.

Calming oils that may be used for Vata
◆ **Sesame oil**

Benefits and effects
1. Settles all the three dosha types and nourishes the body
2. Helps relieve muscular aches, pains and stiffness
3. May prevent hair from turning grey
4. Moisturises dry skin and hair
5. Improves the skin's resilience
6. Warms the body

◆ **Olive oil** is a yellow/green oil extracted from the flesh of the olive. It has a thick consistency and is commonly used in cooking. Extra virgin olive oil is widely available.

Benefits and effects
1. Helps to moisturise skin and hair and so prevents dryness
2. Helps to relieve muscular stiffness and pain
3. Helps to reduce swelling

◆ **Almond oil** is extracted from the kernels of the sweet almond tree. It is a pale yellow oil, rich in nutrients such as unsaturated fatty acids, protein and vitamins A, B, D and E.

Benefits and effects
1. Good to use on clients who have dry hair due to chemical treatments such as colouring or perms

2. Promotes healthy, glossy hair as it stimulates the blood circulation to the scalp
3. Excellent moisturiser for skin and hair
4. Relieves muscular tension, pain and stiffness
5. Warms the body

Cooling oils that may be used for Pita

- **Coconut oil** is a cream-coloured oil extracted from the dried cream of the coconut. The oil is light and has a sweet aroma. At room temperature coconut oil will be solid but will soften when warm. Placing the pot by a radiator or in warm water for a few minutes will warm the oil. Widely used in southern India.

Benefits and effects
1. Softens and moisturises the hair
2. Encourages healthy hair growth and helps to relieve any inflammation
3. Helps the hair to become vibrant and alive

- **Almond oil**
  As above

Warming oils that may be used for Kapa

- **Sesame oil**
  As above
- **Mustard oil** is another popular oil used in India. It has a strong aroma, powerful scent and is thick and yellow in colour. The oil is extracted from the crushed seeds of the mustard plant.

Benefits and effects
1. Stimulates blood circulation to the scalp so helps to promote warmth, therefore is ideal to use in winter months
2. Relieves tension, pain and stiffness in muscles
3. Encourages healthy, glossy hair growth
4. Good to use on people with arthritis

> **REMEMBER**
> Never blend essential oils/herbs/spices with virgin base oils for Shiro-Abhyanga.

Hygiene

The massage therapist needs to have a basic understanding of bacteriology and to be aware of the importance of impeccable cleanliness.

General terms of hygiene

- Antiseptic – substance that inhibits the growth and multiplication of bacteria, e.g. Dettol, Savlon, alcohol
- Asepsis – state of being free of bacteria; the term is used to describe a complete absence of all disease-causing micro-organisms. Articles are said to be aseptic or sterile when they have been treated so that no living pathogenic organism is on or in them
- Disinfectant – substance that is capable of destroying most bacteria, e.g. bleach, surgical spirits
- Disinfection – the term is used to describe the physical or chemical processes by which most pathogenic organisms are destroyed
- Sepsis – state of being infected with bacteria; the term is used to describe a local infective condition resulting from the presence of pus-producing organisms

- Sterilisation – the term is used to describe the process of total destruction of all living micro-organisms

Bacterial infections

Insufficient cleaning or sterilising can allow bacteria to grow and multiply.

- Bacterial infection – a single-cell organism which causes skin disease
- Bacteria are described as:
  1. Non-pathogenic – harmless or friendly bacteria
  2. Pathogenic – disease-causing bacteria
  3. Pathogen – any type of micro-organism that causes bacteria

Symptoms of bacterial infections
- Inflammation
- Redness
- Suppuration (formation of pus)
- Heat

Viral infections

Viruses are minute organisms visible only through an electron microscope. They enter the body though the mouth or skin and through contamination (i.e. water). Viral infections include:

- Influenza
- Herpes simplex
- Herpes zoster
- Hepatitis
- Rubella
- Yellow fever
- Warts

Fungal infections

These are yeast infections and are the most frequent unwelcome guests on our skin. There are five main species:

1. Tine Barbae – affects the bearded areas of the face and neck, hence being restricted to adult males. Ringworm of the beard (barber's itch)
2. Tinea Capitis – affects the scalp. Mainly caught from animals such as cats and dogs
3. Tinea Corpis – affects the trunk and limbs (ringworm)
4. Tinea Cruris – affects the area around the groin and armpits (dhobis itch)
5. Tinea Pedis – affects the area between the toes (athlete's foot)

Insect infestation

As well as the micro-organisms there are two groups of animals which may infest the skin and intestines – insects and worms. Although often irritating and sometimes debilitating, they seldom cause serious disease. They may be difficult to eradicate as the immune system is unable to make antibodies against them. Insect infestation includes scabies, lice and tapeworm.

Cross-infection

The transference of pathogenic micro-organisms from one person to another can be caused by:

Direct contact

As in skin diseases, venereal diseases, oral and respiratory infections

Indirect contact

Via airborne infection, water, food, fomites (clothing, blankets, eating utensils), animals, insects, contaminated instruments, equipment and products

Viral and fungal infections and insect infestations are all very contagious.

All materials and equipment chosen should lend themselves to easy hygiene and maintenance. Check with clients for possible allergies to all equipment in your treatment room.

Table 8.01 *Summary of hygiene procedures*

What	Where	How	Why
Therapist	Overall clean appearance	Personal hygiene	
	Well groomed	Healthy lifestyle	
	In good health	Regular check-ups	
	Cover all cuts	Observing and maintaining professional standards	
		Up-to-date information	Professionalism
			Protection
Client	Suggest shower before treatment	Consultation	Client and therapist confidence
	Cover all cuts	Ensure contraindications do not apply	To avoid cross-infection
	In good health		
Materials and equipment	Towels, oil, oil bottles, trolley, etc.	Sterilisation and disposable	
Premises	Floor, toilets, wash basin, worktops, etc.	Regular cleaning	

Progress Check

1. List five things you could do to ensure the treatment room looks inviting and professional to clients.
2. Name five ways in which you can present a professional image.
3. State five items that may be required in order to carry out an Indian Head Massage treatment.
4. What are the benefits of scalp oil massage?
5. What is meant by the terms 'direct' and 'indirect' cross-infection?

Key Terms

You need to know what these words mean. Go back through the chapter or check in the glossary to find out.

- Healing space
- Ambience
- Professional appearance
- Client care
- Employment standards
- Ethics
- Sacrament
- Beeswax
- Scalp oil massage
- Hygiene
- Cross-infection

Indian Head Massage Techniques and Treatment Areas

After working through this chapter you will be able to:

● Gain a deeper understanding of the different massage techniques

● Recognise the benefits of Indian Head Massage on the upper body

● Describe the beneficial effects of the treatment

● Perform a consultation

● Set up a working area

● Recognise any contraindications

● Recognise medical conditions that could affect the treatment.

Knowing how to be at one with your hands is the core of massage, the one real technique. The more massage you do, the more this knowledge will open itself to you.

Many people first learning massage are nervous, consciously or unconsciously, about the possibility of hurting someone with their hands, and as a result they tend to apply almost no pressure. The pressure you use will vary according to the particular stroke and the part of the body on which it is being used. Working on the client through the clothes will warrant pressure when you offer an Indian Head Massage.

Let the sense of touch be a new form of communication. Relax your hands and keep them as loose and flexible as possible while they are talking to the body. Rough hands will feel abrasive to your client's skin – regularly massage your own hands with oil on a weekly basis. These are the only tools that you need for Indian Head Massage. Make your hands constantly question and listen to the tissues and bones beneath. Tune into the texture of the deeper strata of the muscles. Identify tightness, looseness, thickness or slenderness.

GOOD PRACTICE

Regularly massage and moisturise your hands so they are not rough when you massage.

The effectiveness of most massage strokes depends upon your ability. Certain techniques require that only a specific part of the hands be used to fit the contours of the client's body. Think of ways the stream shapes itself to fit the rocks and hollows in its path.

Maintain an evenness of speed and pressure. Try to eliminate trembling, jerkiness and unnecessary stops and starts. Make any change of either

REMEMBER
Rhythm is an essential ingredient of your massage technique.

speed or pressure a gradual one, never increasing or decreasing too suddenly. Let the movement of your hands be flowing, comfortable and as smooth as possible. You can use different speeds and pressures without sacrificing the steadiness of your movement.

It is a fiction that you have to be physically powerful to apply pressure; use your weight rather than your muscles. Where you need to deliver extra pressure, lean the weight of your upper body through the arms into your hands, rather than by straining with the muscles in your arms and wrists. Straining your muscles will only give you stiff hands, a less flowing quality of movement and a tired back.

Once you have made contact with the client, try not to break it until the treatment has come to an end. Many clients when massaged experience any interruption of physical contact as psychologically distressing. Even when you have to apply oil to the scalp, maintain a link with the client. Bear in mind that your client sitting upright on the chair with the eyes closed will have entered a universe of touch whose one reality is the contact of your hand.

Pay attention to how you are standing, sitting or kneeling. The attention you give to your own comfort will be translated to your client as increased grace and precision in the movement of your hands.

Remember always that you are treating a person and not just an intricate muscle and bone machine. Muscle and bone we are, but human too; and we are human throughout every cubic centimetre of us. Stay aware of this at all times and keep your hands aware of it; it will have a direct and critical influence on the quality of your touch.

REMEMBER
Try to keep as much contact as you can with the client during the massage to ensure it flows smoothly.

Trigun (three) types of touch
Satva indicates harmony and a state of flexibility. A satvic touch is one that is loving, gentle, soft, sensitive and intuitive. It is relaxing, in harmony, balancing and emotionally rejuvenating. It nourishes the nerves, nadis and pranas.

Rajas indicates a state of change, action and movement. It is touch that seeks movement, seeks to open and stimulate. It is very effective to work on the first tissue levels (dhatus), plasma, blood and muscles.

Tamas indicates a state that is blocked, stuck or held – as in a belief. A tamasic touch is one that opens and liberates. It is deep, strong and penetrating.

Indian Head Massage techniques
The techniques used in Indian Head Massage are simple and effective and are a combination of the following range of massage movements.

Effleurage
A movement which is mainly done with a flat palm and fingers of both hands close together. It is a rhythmic movement which should conform to the normal contours of the client's body.

REMEMBER
Effleurer is a French word meaning to touch lightly.

The movement must always follow the direction of venous return (blood in veins) back to the heart, and also in the direction of lymphatic drainage towards a group of lymph nodes. The hands stay in contact with the body during the return of the stroke.

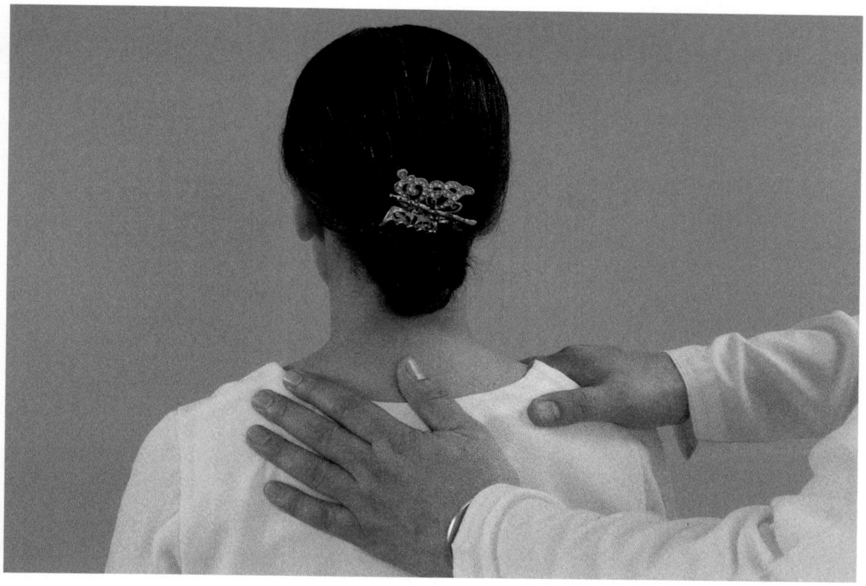

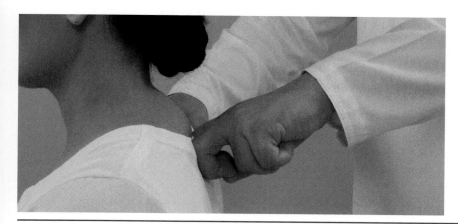

Fig. 9.01 *Effleurage massage movement*

Use of effleurage

- Introduces the therapist's touch
- To spread the massage medium (when used) so that the whole area is lubricated
- Used after stronger and stimulating strokes to soothe
- Helps to attain a sense of continuity in treatment by linking one movement to the next
- Slow and rhythmical strokes help client to relax

Effects of effleurage

- Calming, soothing and sedative
- Improves blood circulation and increases lymphatic flow to assist the elimination of waste products and circulation
- Aids desquamation (removal of dead skin cells) so the skin will look healthier and feel smoother
- Improves general circulation by increasing blood flow in veins

Movements related to effleurage

- Stroking – calming effect with slow and gentle strokes
- Superficial effleurage – relaxing effect with slow and firm strokes
- Deep effleurage – stimulating effect with quicker and firmer strokes

Frictions

Fig. 9.02 *Friction massage movement*

Frictions consist of small deep movements and is mainly used on localised areas on thickening in muscles, and around tendons or ligaments.

Frictions should cause the skin to rub against structures underlying it, so that one layer of tissue is pressed firmly against another with steady pressure, maintained throughout.

Movements are performed in a circular or oblique direction with the palmar surface of the hand, fingers or thumbs.

Uses of frictions
- Provides deep localised massage to connective tissue
- Breaks down fibrosistic or arthritic adhesions
- Stimulates nerves

Effects of frictions
- Stimulates the circulation, thereby bringing oxygen and nutrients to the area worked and producing erythema (redness)
- Can have an invigorating and refreshing effect through the stimulation of the spinal nerves and sympathetic nerves, if worked on the spine area
- Localised hyperaemia helps to nourish joint structures and increase and maintain joint mobility

Movements related to frictions
- Circular friction
- Transverse friction (i.e. across the grain)
- Knuckling

Tapotement

Tapotement movements are, in general, rhythmical, stimulating and fast. The hands usually work alternately and the wrists are kept flexible. The movements are performed either with cupped hands, with the ulnar surface of the hands, fingers or loose fists. All movements should be light, springy and stimulating, and should not cause pain or bruising.

Tapotement movements are also known as percussion movements. All tapotement movements are stimulating and so are usually omitted from a relaxing type of massage. The area worked is rapidly stroked using alternate hands.

Uses of tapotement
- Helps to improve and strengthen muscle tone
- Aids the breakdown of fatty deposits
- Creates heat

Effects of tapotement
- Deep, stimulating and refreshing effect on nerve endings
- Increases circulation to the area so that erythema is produced
- Helps to improve circulation and increases absorption of nutrients
- Helps with the elimination of waste products in tissues and muscles
- Breaks down and mobilises fatty deposits
- Tones and strengthens sagging muscles

REMEMBER
Tapoter is a French word meaning to tap.

REMEMBER
Tapotement movements are also known as percussion movements.

- Increases blood flow to the lungs and thorax, loosening mucus and easing congestion for a better interchange of gases, when performed on the back

Movements related to tapotement
- Beating – skin is struck with hands held in a loose fist
- Cupping – hands cupped
- Flaying – skin is struck with stretched fingers
- Hacking – skin is struck with the ulnar surface of hands, with fingers relaxed – if not the movement becomes a karate chop and this would be most undesirable!

Hacking

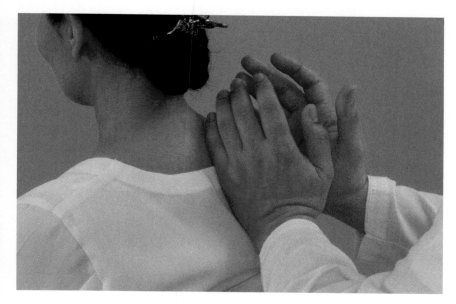

Fig. 9.03 *Hacking massage movement*

A stimulating tapotement movement, hacking is movement which is very invigorating and can stimulate a lethargic client. Hacking can help in toning muscles. It is done using a very relaxed rhythm with the sides of the palms.

Uses of hacking
- To revive someone who is falling asleep
- To get one's mind back into one's body
- To bring about control and movement in tissue and increase blood flow

Effects of hacking
- Revival of senses of the person being hacked
- Stimulates circulation of the skin and also relaxes the muscles
- Improve sluggish lymphatic circulation

Movements related to hacking
- Using the sides of the hands alternately
- Chop-chop movements
- Keep hands in relaxed mode

Fig. 9.04 *Pétrissage massage movement*

Pétrissage

These movements either press the muscle onto the bone or lift the muscle away from the bone. The whole hand, fingers or thumbs can be used. Pétrissage movements are deeper movements in which soft tissues are compressed.

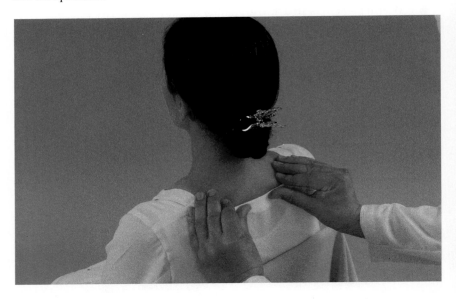

Uses of pétrissage
- Helps to soften fat by creating warmth
- Generates heat and therefore hyperaemia in tissue
- Performed quickly and slowly to stimulate and relax the underlying structure worked on

Effects of pétrissage
- Blood and lymphatic circulation is increased, encouraging fresh oxygen and nutrients to be delivered to the tissues and an increased removal of waste products
- Erythema is produced
- Helps to remove lactic acid in the circulation, alleviating stiffness and refreshing muscles
- Speeds up the elimination of toxins
- Increases the secretion of sebum, so moisturises skin and hair
- Increases the rate of cellular exchange
- Flattens, broadens or stretches tissues

Movement related to pétrissage
- Picking up (pinching) – the tissues are picked up and lifted away from the bone and then released
- Kneading (squeezing) –– the muscle is pressed onto the bone using firm movements. It can be performed with one hand or both hands, or with the palm, fingers and/or thumbs
- Skin rolling
- Wringing

Vibrations

The hands or fingers, usually of one hand, are vibrated so that a fine tremor is produced in the tissues. The tremor is produced by the contraction of the forearm muscles.

Uses of vibrations

- Stimulates sluggish lymphatic drainage
- Relieves tension and so induces relaxation

Effects of vibrations

- Promotes relaxation to the muscles and is soothing to nerves
- Relieves pain and fatigue
- Relieves tiredness and lethargy

Marma points

Massage techniques that address the marma points should be incorporated during Indian Head Massage treatments. Applying pressure to the marma points treats the client holistically.

Uses of working on marma points

- Stimulating marma points by massage can bring healing effects to a specific area of the mind-body structure.

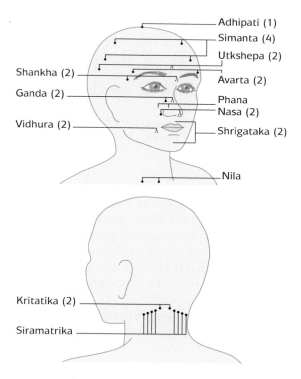

Fig. 9.05 *Marma points*

Effects of working on marma points

- Stimulation of these points promotes physical and mental rehabilitation for stroke victims, general weakness, musco-skeletal aches and pains and stress.
- By applying pressure at the Marma points in a systematic way, relief and cure transcends the recipient.

Movements related to marma points

- All marma points are very sensitive areas. Hence massage at these vital points should be done gently, by using the pad of the thumb and fingers. These points are, more importantly, used for stimulating internal organs and systems of the body.
- Marma points should be touched with great care. Massage using sesame oil, rubbing in a compact anti-clockwise direction gradually increasing your pressure, then in a clockwise direction, gradually releasing your pressure.

REMEMBER
Marma points are sensitive areas and so massage to them should be gentle.

Treatment areas

Upper back and shoulders

- Tension is often experienced in the shoulder girdle.
- The shoulders are designed for flexibility and movement.
- Tension in this area will result in a loss of flexibility. This will have an immediate effect on the body in that it restricts the ribs and how deeply we breathe. It slows down circulation, creates headaches and the body feels out of balance.
- Massage in this area can help to eliminate muscle tension and improve joint mobility.

Arms and hands

- People carry a lot of tension in their hands and arms due to their constant use.
- Many people are involved in tasks that cause repetitive strain injuries to their arms and hands, which can lead to, for example, carpal tunnel syndrome.
- Frequent actions are holding and clutching as well as lifting heavy objects.
- It is very relaxing to counteract these movements by massaging the arms, hands, palms and fingers.

Neck

- The neck is a strong, complex region where the skeletal and muscular systems allow the head free movement.
- Poor posture creates an imbalance and can cause the neck muscles to tense up. This results in the neck muscles becoming permanently contracted, causing tightness and congestion, reducing neck mobility and often resulting in headache and eyestrain.
- The head is designed to balance upon the neck vertebrae without strain.
- Massage in this area helps lymph drainage, eliminates muscle tension, stimulates circulation and improves mobility.

Scalp and face

- The skull is covered by a thin layer of muscles which tighten when we are tense, resulting in headaches and feelings of anxiety.
- Tension also gathers in the face causing the scalp, eye, jaw and mouth region to tighten. This can result in such things as headaches, hair loss, eyestrain, and neck and shoulder problems.
- Tension in the temple region constricts the flow of blood. This can lead to headaches and eyestrain but also to the hair turning grey around the temples as the hair roots are starved of nutrients.

- Massage to the scalp and face stimulates and improves scalp circulation and improves the strength, texture and growth of hair. It soothes and rebalances energy flow, creating a feeling of calm and wellbeing.
- Ayurvedic facial rejuvenation (not part of IHM) is a light massage specially designed to improve functioning of the lymphatic system.

Ears

- Ears are extremely important in an Indian Head Massage treatment. According to oriental medicine there are 108 points on the ear alone.
- Known indications are irritations in the ear, frontal and paranasal sinuses, sinusitis, rhinitis, co-ordination of the cerebral hemispheres, noises in the ears (ringing), activation of the blood flow, the metabolic process and lymphatic system.

Hair and skin

- Ayurveda emphasises the all-important value of a good diet, as it creates good quality nourishment (rasa), which in turn will nourish the blood (rakta) and subsequently influence the skin.
- Science of life declares that skin diseases occur primarily due to sluggish liver function, which leads to pita and kapa dosha dysfunction. Another vital factor that contributes to healthy appearance is a clean bowel. Hence the need for regular and complete bowel evacuation.
- The hair is the metabolic end product of bone and marrow. Thus if the diet falls short of nourishing bones, the quantity of hair is affected. Similarly stress and worry leads to unhealthy hair. A wholesome diet is necessary for good skin and hair. Ayurvedic skin- and hair-care products are formulated with these facts in mind during examination.

Progress Check

1. What are the three types of touch?
2. What is effleurage?
3. What are the uses and effects of pétrissage?
4. What is the difference between friction and vibration movements?
5. What are the benefits of working on marma points?

Key Terms

You need to know what these words mean. Go back through the chapter or check in the glossary to find out.

- Trigun
- Effleurage
- Pétrissage
- Tapotement
- Friction
- Vibrations
- Marma points

Indian Head Massage Treatment Sequence

After working through this chapter you will be able to:

- Demonstrate the classical massage movements: effleurage, frictions, kneading, pétrissage, tapotement, vibrations
- Perform a treatment on a fully clothed client with or without oils
- Demonstrate a high standard of hygiene and professionalism at all times
- Complete the treatment in a commercially acceptable time
- Recommend appropriate post-treatment advice
- Communicate effectively with a wide range of clients
- Practise the treatment on a variety of clients in a multiplicity of situations.

Shiro-Abhyanga is for reconnecting tissues, stimulating metabolism, expelling toxins, increasing digestive function, relieving muscular tension, breaking up knots and treating rheumatoid diseases and arthritis. Clients need to be calmed, pacified, nourished and nurtured.

The foundation of every technique is silence. The stillness of mind is the fundamental element needed for a successful Indian Head Massage. Stillness allows the technique to flow uninhibited from you, enabling you to merge with your client. In this state, prana flows effortlessly to your client. This quality some call love, some call it the divine. Whatever the name, this grace can only happen when there is silence.

Perhaps the most important technique is preparing the client for the therapy session. This is often overlooked, yet it is fundamental in any therapeutic situation. The failure to properly prepare your client mentally, emotionally and physically will reduce or nullify the effectiveness of your treatment. Proper preparation will enhance the effectiveness of the treatment.

The reasons for this are as complicated as clients vary from culture to culture. Yet it can be summarised simply that every person is looking for love. Each of us needs to feel cared for and secure before embarking on any kind of therapeutic transformation. But before this process of transformation can happen, the client must feel – at least intuitively – safe and secure. This is the basic environment that you must provide.

> **REMEMBER**
> If your mind is distracted, your treatment will not succeed.

If your mind and pranas are distracted your treatment will not succeed, even though your physical movements may follow a routine. The therapist should remain centred and focused on the client. The Indian Head Massage technique requires the therapist to be energetic and firm. A silent mind aids this by allowing the pranas to move out freely. Clockwise circular movements bring prana into the body and anti-clockwise movements liberate trapped energy from the body. This also helps to open, liberate and stimulate the plasma, lymphatic system and blood circulation, and nourish the skin.

> **REMEMBER**
> The therapist should remain centred and focused on the client throughout the treatment.

Fig. 10.1 *Equipment*

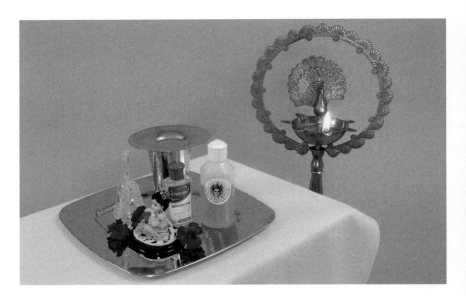

Next there is the physical preparation. This relies on your professional skill to use the consultation and your observations to measure the client's overall strength and their openness to you and your work. Failure to understand this can put you in an embarrassing or uncomfortable position. Or you can throw your own failure back onto the client with remarks like: 'you didn't let go' or 'pain is part of the process' or 'those knots sure didn't want to go, but I managed'. These are all examples of how therapists avoid their own responsibility and fail to understand their client and their capability to receive the treatment. Indian Head Massage is far more effective, especially in the long run, when this is understood.

The technique should begin with your own harmony, as whatever you are goes directly into the client. It is best to begin with five minutes of nam-simran before working on the client. When you are centred and calm, protect your treatment space and yourself, then begin.

After having carried out the consultation process, remove the client's shoes/boots and place them outside the practice room. Wrap your client's feet in a large warm towel and place them on a footstool or a large cushion. Ask to be excused to wash your hands, then activate your hand chakras.

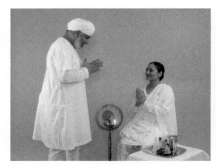

Fig. 10.02 *Welcoming the client*

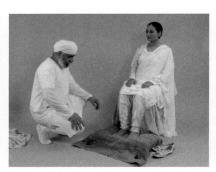

Fig. 10.03 *Preparing the client for treatment*

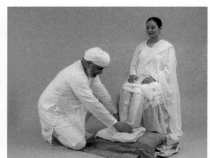

Fig. 10.04 *Wrapping the client's feet in a towel*

Wrap your client's feet in a warm towel and place them on a large cushion.

Always speak softly and clearly – your tone of voice and manner should reflect a genuine feeling of caring and consideration towards your client. Check for comfort, warmth and pressure. In the delivery of the treatment keep a continual assessment on the suppleness of the regions that you have worked on. A professional is someone who can do his best work when he doesn't feel like it.

Always speak softly and clearly to your client, and always listen carefully to what she has to say.

Shiro-Abhyanga – traditional Indian Head Massage sequence

Prerequisites

- Client care
- Consultation
- Remove all hair clips/adornments
- Ask clients to arrive with clean hair free of hairspray and gels.
- Check your pressure after half a dozen movements or so.
- Wash hands with an antiseptic hand wash.
- Activate your hand chakras.
- Always make sure that your instructions follow your actions.
- Protect yourself, shake your body to loosen up and gently enter the client's aura.
- Take a minute to gently shake out your whole body. This is especially important if you are staying in one position for any length of time.
- Start with the hands and feet, then legs, arms and the whole body including the head. It helps loosen stiff muscles and allows energy to flow freely again.
- Keep your knees slightly bent, which maintains body stability.
- Only work as far as the back of the chair will comfortably allow you to do so.
- Keeping your elbows bent during the treatment reduces the strain on your shoulder joints.
- All movements are simultaneous unless otherwise indicated.
- Say hello to the body – a gentle introduction of your touch to the client. Remain in touch with the client's body until treatment has come to an end.

> **REMEMBER**
> Carrying out five minutes of nam-simran before working on a client will help to prepare you for giving the treatment.

Upper back and shoulders

Step 1

Part 1

Stand behind the client, place your hands on her shoulders and ask the client to close her eyes and take three deep breaths.

Part 2

Place your hands on the client's head and take three deep breaths to synchronise your breathing with that of the client.

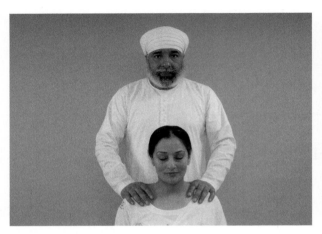

Fig. 10.05 *Step 1, Part 1*

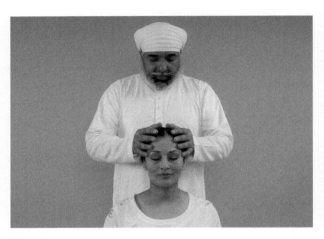

Fig. 10.06 *Step 1, Part 2*

Step 2

Effleurage each side of the client's upper back and across the shoulder girdle three times each side. Always work on the left side of the client with your left hand and support the client with your right hand. Repeat the movement on the opposite side of the client.

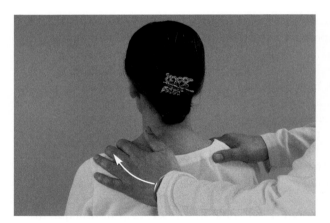

Fig. 10.07 *Step 2*

Step 3

Thumb sweeping – standing behind the client, deliver a sequence of three movements. With your fingers on the client's shoulders, reach down with your thumbs and place them as far as they can go either side of the spine.

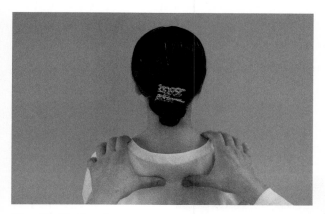

Fig. 10.08 *Step 3*

Part 1

Move thumbs upwards then outwards to meet your little finger at the corner of the shoulder girdle. Repeat three times.

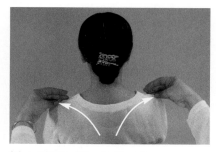

Fig. 10.09 *Step 3, Part 1*

Part 2

Repeat as above (half way along the shoulder girdle) by allowing the thumbs to move up and out to meet your middle finger. Repeat three times.

Part 3

As above, but let the thumbs move up to meet your index finger at the neck. Repeat three times.

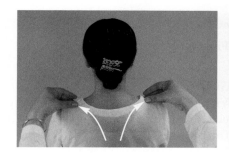

Fig. 10.10 *Part 2*

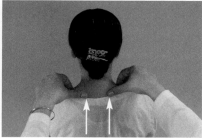

Fig. 10.11 *Part 3*

Step 4

Part 1

Heel of hand rub – stand at the client's right side. With the heel of your left hand rub anti-clockwise from the client's left shoulder edge along to the neck, and then down between the shoulder blade and the spine. Then, in a clockwise direction, move the heel of your hand up to the neck and along the shoulder girdle to finish at the corner of the shoulder. Repeat three times.

Part 2

Repeat as above but on the client's right side, working with your right hand.

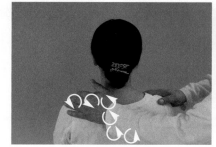

Fig. 10.12 *Step 4, Part 1*

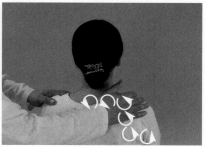

Fig. 10.13 *Part 2*

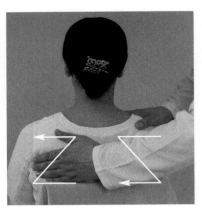

Fig. 10.14 *Step 5*

Step 5

Part 1

Finger frictions – stand at the client's right side. With all fingers of your left hand extended, rub vigorously sideways, following the shape of a Z, on the client's left upper back. Follow the Z shape back up to where you had started. Repeat three times.

Part 2

Repeat as above but on the client's right side, working with your right hand.

Step 6

Effleurage (as in step 2) each side of the client's upper back and across the shoulder girdle, three times each side.

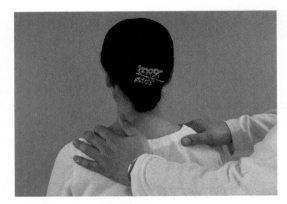

Fig. 10.15 *Step 6*

Step 7

Vibrate – with the knuckles of your right-hand index and middle fingers either side of the client's spine, work down gently between each vertebra from T1 as far down as the chair will allow. Work back up to T1 with the knuckles of your left hand. Repeat three times.

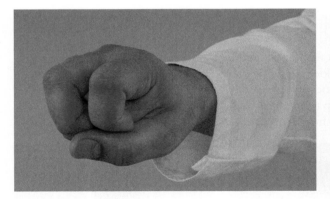

Fig. 10.16 *Step 7*

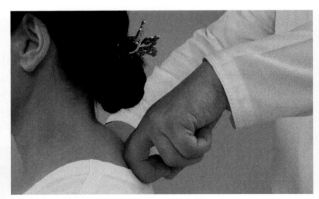

Fig. 10.17 *Step 7*

GOOD PRACTICE

Don't forget to watch your posture throughout the treatment to help avoid getting aches and pains.

Step 8

Part 1

Thumb pushes – standing behind the client, place the palms of your hands at the corners of the client's shoulders, with thumbs resting above shoulder blades. Push your thumbs (nail pointing forward), applying medium pressure, up and over the shoulder. Repeat three times. The movement should be similar to that of closing a honey-jar lid.

REMEMBER
In – means movements coming in towards the neck from the shoulders.

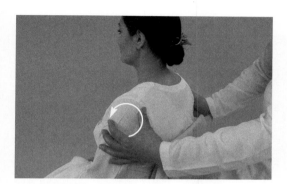

Fig. 10.18 *Step 8, Part 1*

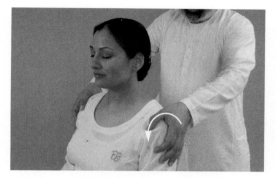

Fig. 10.19 *Step 8, Part 1*

Part 2

Repeat the above movement at the middle of the client's shoulders, three times.

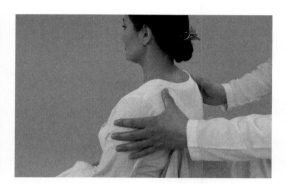

Fig. 10.20 *Step 8, Part 2*

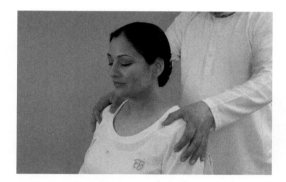

Fig. 10.21 *Step 8, Part 2*

Part 3

Repeat at the junction of the client's neck and shoulders, three times.

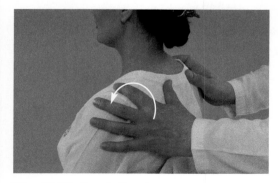

Fig. 10.22 *Step 8, Part 3*

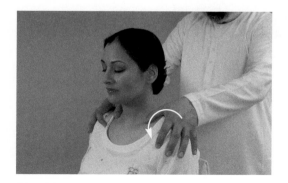

Fig. 10.23 *Step 8, Part 3*

Step 9

Part 1

Finger pulls – standing behind the client, anchor your thumbs either side of the spine with your fingers in front of the shoulders, near the base of the neck. Pull your fingers back towards your thumbs. Repeat three times.

Part 2

Repeat at the middle of the client's shoulders three times.

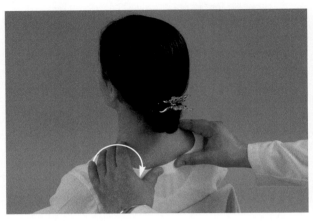

Fig. 10.24 *Step 9, Part 1*

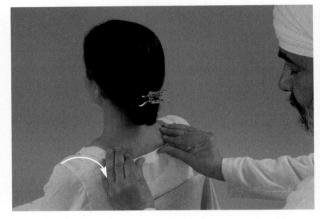

Fig. 10.25 *Part 2*

Part 3

Repeat further along, near the corners of the client's shoulders three times.

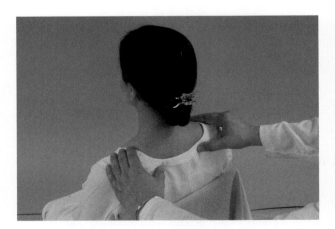

Fig. 10.26 *Part 3*

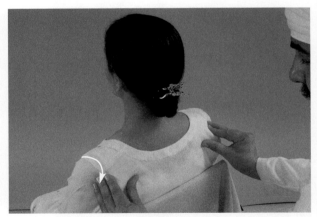

Fig. 10.27 *Part 3*

Step 10

Part 1

Heel pushes – standing behind the client, use the heels of your hands to push over the trapezius shoulder muscles. Begin from furthest away from the neck and repeat three times.

Part 2

Repeat at the middle of the client's shoulders three times.

Part 3

Repeat at the shoulders, near the base of the client's neck, three times.

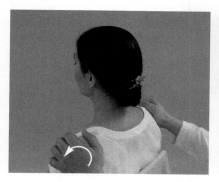

Fig. 10.28 *Step 10, Part 1*

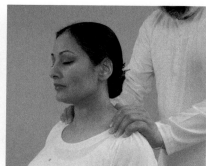

Fig. 10.29 *Part 2*

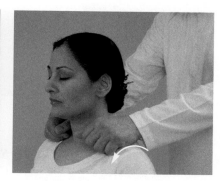

Fig. 10.30 *Part 3*

Step 11

Part 1

Pick up and hold – standing behind the client, place the heel of your hands near the base of the client's neck. Pick up the trapezius shoulder muscles and hold with medium pressure, then release. Repeat three times.

Part 2

Repeat at the middle of the client's shoulders three times.

Part 3

Repeat at the corners of the client's shoulders three times.

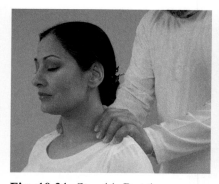

Fig. 10.31 *Step 11, Part 1*

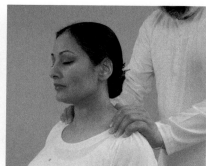

Fig. 10.32 *Part 2*

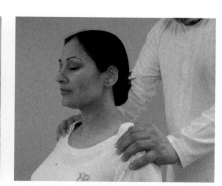

Fig. 10.33 *Part 3*

Step 12

Smoothing with your forearms – standing behind the client, gently sweep from the client's neck to theend of the shoulders three times, maintaining equal pressure, speed and rhythm on both sides.

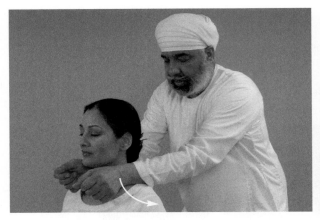

Fig. 10.34 *Step 12*

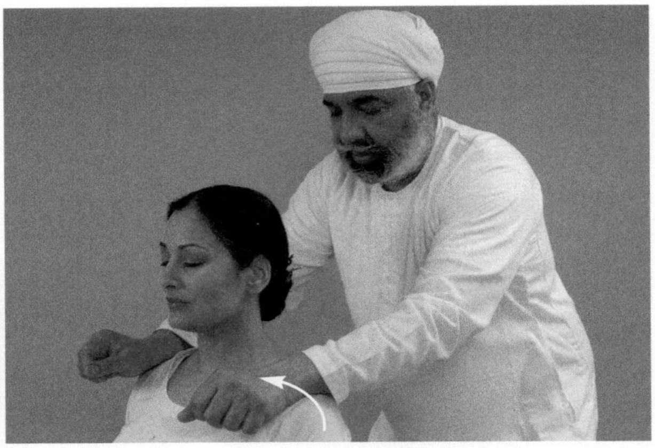

Fig. 10.35 *Step 12*

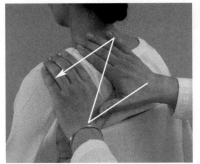

Fig. 10.36 *Step 13*

Step 13

Chopping (pinching) – kneeling or sitting behind the client, with both palms of your hands resting completely against the client's entire upper back, slightly raise the heel of your right hand so that the index fingers of both hands create the pinching movement.

Start from the client's left shoulder and follow the figure of a squashed 'Z' and then back up three times.

Step 14

Hacking – standing behind the client, work from the left shoulder, skipping the spine, to the right shoulder and back three times (move along the shoulder girdle only).

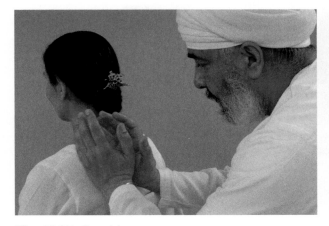

Fig. 10.37 *Step 14*

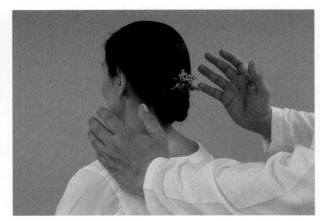

Fig. 10.38 *Step 14*

Step 15

Part 1

Gentle pick up and hold three times (as in step 11) – standing behind the client, place the palms of your hands at the corners of the client's shoulder with the heel of your hand behind the shoulders and your fingers in front. Pick up the client's trapezius shoulder muscles and hold with medium pressure, then release. Repeat three times.

Part 2

Repeat at the middle of the client's shoulders three times.

Part 3

Repeat at the base of the client's shoulders, three times.
Assess if the shoulder girdle region has become supple, compared to when you started.

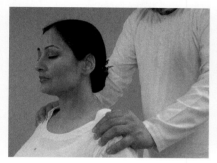 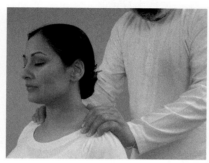 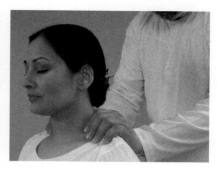

Fig. 10.39 *Step 15, Part 1*   **Fig. 10.40** *Part 2*   **Fig. 10.41** *Part 3*

Step 16

Effleurage (as in step 2) each side of the upper back and across the shoulders, three times each side.

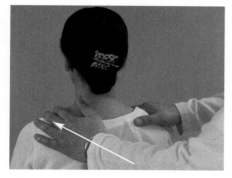

Fig. 10.42 *Step 16*

Step 17

While standing behind the client, hold your hands on their shoulders to finish.

Benefits

- After holding a stretched posture, the muscles of the shoulders naturally relax, balancing the position of the shoulder girdle. Breathing will become deeper and easier. Sometimes the client receiving the massage will sigh or take a very long, deep breath. This type of breath is a good sign of deep release.
- Hidden tension that accumulates around the shoulders will have been released. This is most common among clients who sit at desks and work with computers or long-distance vehicle drivers.

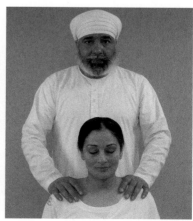

Fig. 10.43 *Step 17*

Arms

Step 1
Part 1
Compressing – kneel or sit at the side of your client. Butterfly-clasp your fingers and, using the palms of your hands, squash the top of the client's left/right upper arm, posterior and anterior. Repeat three times.

Part 2
Repeat half way down the client's upper right arm three times.

Part 3
Repeat just above the client's elbow of the right arm three times.

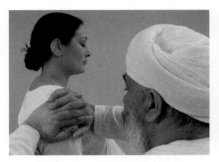

Fig. 10.44 *Step 1, Part 1*

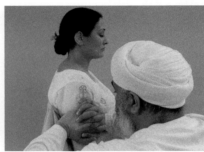

Fig. 10.45 *Part 2*

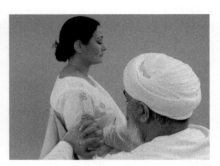

Fig. 10.46 *Part 3*

Step 2
Part 1
Gentle squeeze – still kneeling or sitting at the side of your client, anchor your fingers at the inner surface of the top of the client's right arm and use the heels of your hand to squeeze the outer surface of the arm. Work from the deltoid muscle to the palm with medium pressure. Repeat three times.

Part 2
Gentle squeeze – repeat half way down the client's upper right arm, three times.

Part 3
Gentle squeeze – repeat above the elbow of the client's right arm, three times.

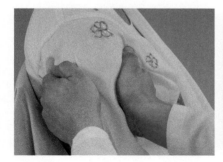

Fig. 10.47 *Step 2, Part 1*

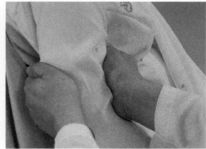

Fig. 10.48 *Part 2*

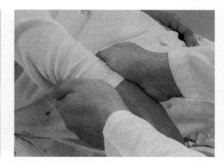

Fig. 10.49 *Part 3*

Step 3

Part 1

Hold the Aman point located between the client's thumb and index finger on the right hand, while kneeling or sitting at the side of the client.

While maintaining a firm hold of the client's Aman point, use your right hand and press your thumb on the top of the client's hand, against your index and middle fingers, on the palm of the client's hand.

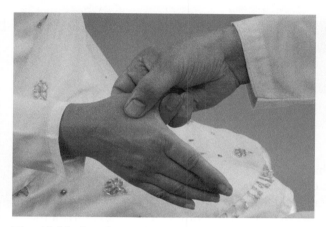

Fig. 10.50 *Step 3, Part 1*

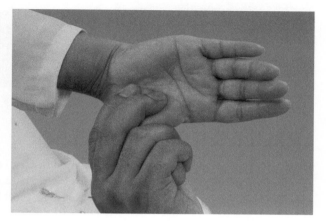

Fig. 10.51 *Step 3, Part 1*

Part 2

Massage each finger and thumb three times, starting with the little finger. Hold the finger between the thumb and index finger of your right hand and quickly work down to the top of the nail. The next movement slides down the sides of the same finger. Repeat a third time on the top of the finger again. As you finish each movement, gently flick or snap your fingers to release stagnant prana.

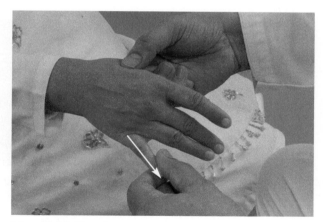

Fig. 10.52 *Part 2*

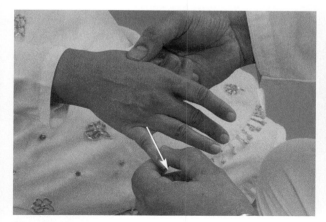

Fig. 10.53 *Part 2*

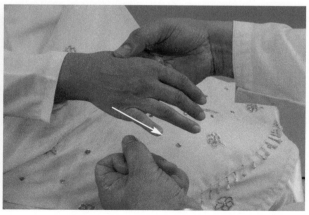

Fig. 10.54 *Part 2*

Part 3

Finger lock – with your right hand, hold the client's right arm just above the wrist. Rotate the client's wrist anti-clockwise and clockwise three times with your right hand, finishing with a wrist stretch. Repeat three times.

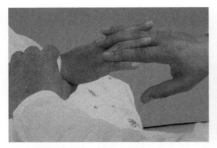

Fig. 10.55 *Part 3*

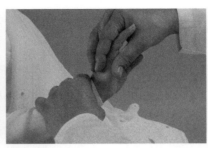

Fig. 10.56 *Part 3*

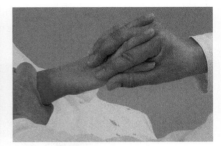

Fig. 10.57 *Part 3*

Part 4

Turn your hand so that the client's palm is facing up, and activate the client's hand chakras on the palms and fingertips. Rest the client's right hand on your right hand and, with the tip of your right-hand thumb, rotate anti-clockwise and clockwise three times each at the centre of the client's palm. Repeat with the pads of all fingers and thumb.

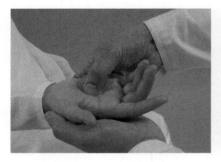

Fig. 10.58 *Part 4 (palm chakra)*

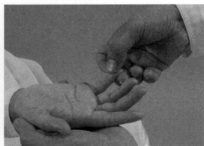

Fig. 10.59 *Part 4 (finger chakras)*

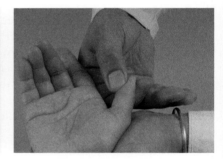

Fig. 10.60 *Part 4 (thumb chakras)*

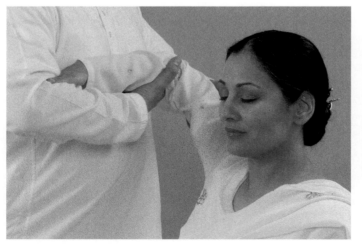

Fig. 10.61 *Step 4*

Step 4

Gently mobilise each shoulder – stand at the client's right side and support the forearm in your left forearm. Make sure the client's hand rests in your elbow and, with your left hand, mobilise the shoulder joint anti-clockwise and clockwise three times. The bigger the circle you make with the client's elbow, the superior the movement.

Step 5

Repeat steps 1, 2, 3 and 4 on the client's left arm.

Step 6

Part 1

Heel roll – standing behind the client, place your hands on top of both deltoid muscles, fingers at the front of the arms, heels behind. Roll the heels over the muscles to meet your fingertips. Repeat three times. Make sure that you work within the client's comfort zone.

Part 2

Repeat at the middle of the client's upper arms three times.

Part 3

Repeat just above the client's elbows three times.

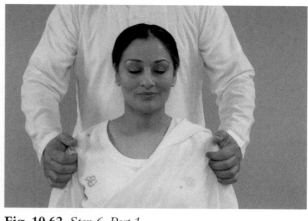

Fig. 10.62 *Step 6, Part 1*

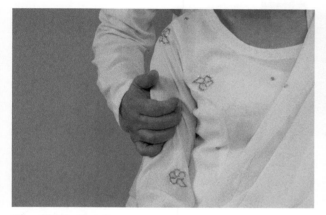

Fig. 10.63 *Part 2*

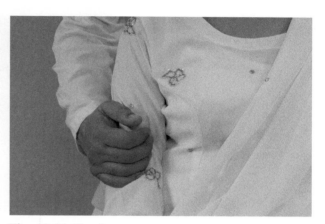

Fig. 10.64 *Part 3*

Step 7

Shoulder lift – with the client's arms securely folded, place your hands under their elbows. Instruct the client to take a deep breath in and pull the elbows up. Instruct the client to breathe out, and push the elbows down gently. Repeat three times. This technique is designed to re-train the shoulder muscles to relax. Always make sure that your actions follow your instructions.

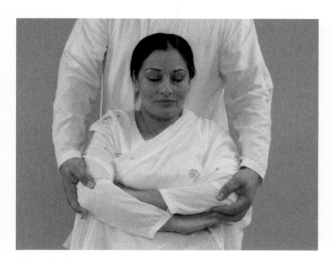

Fig. 10.65 *Step 7*

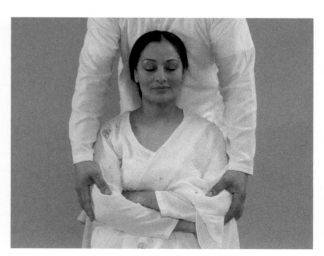

Fig. 10.66 *Step 7*

Step 8

Smoothing with your forearms – standing behind the client, gently sweep from the neck to the elbows. Repeat three times, maintaining equal pressure, speed and rhythm on both sides.

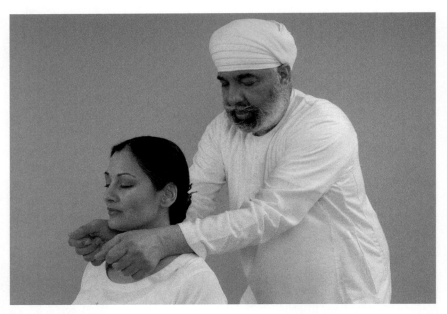

Fig. 10.67 *Step 8*

Benefits

- Benefits wrist injuries, inflammation, stiff finger joints, tennis or stiff elbow, metabolic problems, cramps in upper arm, poor circulation of blood to hand, pain in neck and shoulders, shoulder weakness, frozen shoulder, numbness in hands, difficulty in finger movements.

Neck

Step 1

Part 1

Rock – stand at the client's side, place one hand on her forehead and the other hand at the back of the scalp. Gently rock the head forwards and backwards to release tension. Repeat three times.

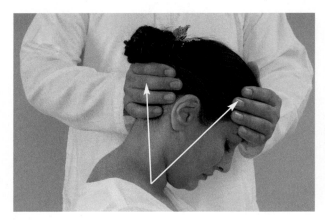

Fig. 10.68 *Step 1, Part 1*

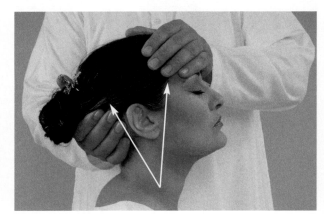

Fig. 10.69 *Step 1, Part 1*

Attempt to get the client's chin to touch the chest, and the back of the head to comfortably drop behind the shoulder girdle. This is best done in a sequence of gentle stretch movements of the neck, i.e.

- 20° forward and 20° back,
- 40° forward and 40° back, then
- 60° forwards and 60° back.

The most difficult part of the human anatomy to be placed in someone else's hands is the head. Clients are almost giving you control of all their senses, so provide your client with confidence in your movements. Always place your working hand behind the scalp as it will reassure you of your client's poise. Roll head from the base of the neck and not from the atlas.

Step 2

Neck flexion and extension (roll) – stand behind the client. Place your hands on either side of the client's head and gently roll the head and neck three times anti-clockwise and clockwise.

Spread your fingers and hold the head firmly so that it does not escape from your hands. In your rotation, attempt to touch the client's chin to their chest, the left ear to their left shoulder, comfortably lean the head towards the back, and the right ear to the right shoulder. Do not place your hands over the client's ears!

The delicate muscles of the neck respond to simple stretching. The neck moves in three different motions. Tilting the head forward is called neck flexion, moving it side to side is called lateral neck flexion, and leaning the head backward is called extension.

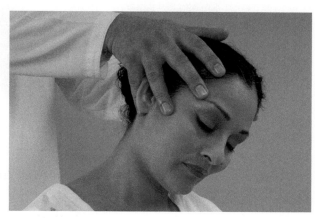

Fig. 10.70 *Step 2*

Step 3

Turn – hold the client's head securely in the upright position. Gently turn the head so the nose is looking over the left shoulder. Repeat slowly, turning the head so the nose is over the right shoulder. You need to turn in each direction once only so that you can assess the mobility of the neck.

Adjustment – if movement is restricted in one direction a correction may be made. Have the client turn her head to the direction that was not restricted and place your hand firmly against her forehead on that side. Instruct the client to take a deep breath and hold it for a count of ten while pushing against your hand. Repeat the head turns to demonstrate improvement of mobility. Do this correction only once time during each treatment.

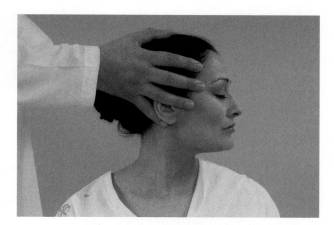

Fig. 10.71 *Step 3*

GOOD PRACTICE

Always move your client's head slowly and smoothly to avoid possible injury.

Step 4

Grasp and pull back posterior (back of the neck) – stand at the side of the client, with one hand supporting the forehead, and tilt the head slightly forward with the other hand. Spread the thumb and fingers either side of the base of the neck and pull back to meet at the spine, using firm contact with the skin. Repeat three times.

Repeat half way up the neck three times.

Repeat at the top of the neck three times.

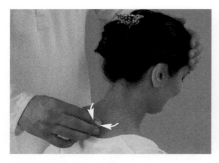

Fig. 10.72 *Step 4*

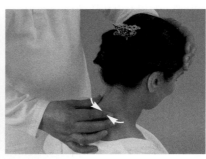

Fig. 10.73 *Step 4*

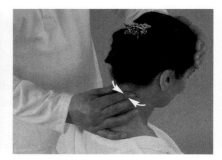

Fig. 10.74 *Step 4*

Step 5

Vibrations – standing behind the client, cross your index fingers so they sit on top of the middle finger. Vibrate with your middle finger from the base of neck to occiput and slide down. Repeat three times.

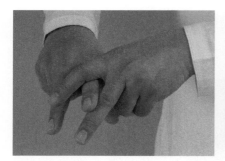

Fig. 10.75 *Step 5*

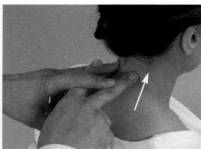

Fig. 10.76 *Step 5*

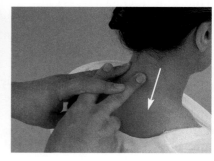

Fig. 10.77 *Step 5*

Step 6

Stand at the side of your client and support the occiput with one hand. Spread the thumb and middle finger of your other hand underneath the collarbone to meet at the sternum, then gently rotate the tips of your thumb and middle finger anti-clockwise and clockwise three times on the nila marma points. When rotating, focus your attention on your wrist and both the thumb and middle finger will move in the same direction.

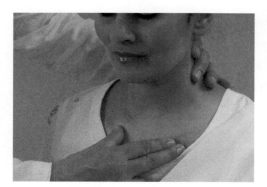

Fig. 10.78 *Step 6*

Step 7

Stand at the side of the client and support the occiput with one hand. Hook your thumb and middle finger, with the index finger of your other hand between them, at the side of the client's neck into the mandibular bone where the manya marma points lie. This action will stimulate the thymus gland, which will boost the immune system.

Step 8

Stand at the side of the client and support the head with one hand. From the windpipe, slide your thumb and middle finger underneath the mandible (lower jaw bone) to meet the chin. With your middle finger resting under the tip of the mandible, and thumb tucked in at the centre of the chin crease, gently rotate anti-clockwise and clockwise three times.

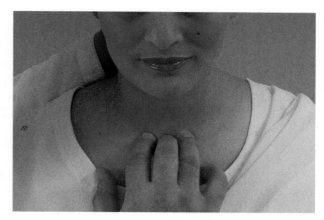

Fig. 10.79 *Step 7*

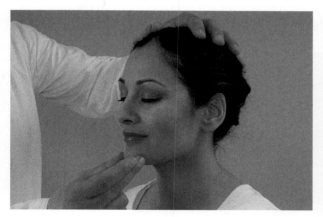

Fig. 10.80 *Step 8*

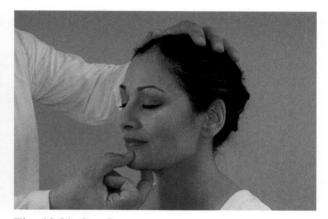

Fig. 10.81 *Step 8*

Benefits
- Clears chest congestion
- Improves the tone of the voice
- Assists the balance of the thyroid and parathyroid functions
- Releases neck tension which initiates a relaxation response in the whole body by opening up the flow of prana from the spine
- Balances the electromagnetic energies of the front and the back of the brain. This can help bring deeply buried memories to the conscious mind and release them
- Balances feelings of anger, pride and frustration
- Helps to regulate blood sugar
- Moderates mood swings
- Improves digestion

> **REMEMBER**
> All marma points should be touched with great care, rubbing in compact anti-clockwise circles, gradually increasing pressure, and in a clockwise direction, slowly releasing pressure.

Step 9
Tilt head.

For the next four movements, stand behind the client. Tilt the client's head to one side by placing your right palm on her forehead, resting your right elbow on her right shoulder girdle and allowing your right hand to take the weight of her head. (The average head weighs around 5.5 kg.)

At this point, moisten your thumb and fingertips with warm sesame massage oil. Warm oil is more soothing and relaxing and penetrates the skin better. It also deepens the effect of the massage by nourishing the muscle tissue and lubricating the layers of connective tissue. Be careful not to use too much oil as it may escape onto the client's clothes and shoulders. Use a very small amount of oil to allow your fingers to flow easily over the client's skin.

REMEMBER
Warm oil is more smoothing and relaxing and penetrates the skin better than cool oil.

Step 10
Part 1
Friction – using all the fingers of your left hand, work from the base of the neck and up to the occipital bone, thirteen times.

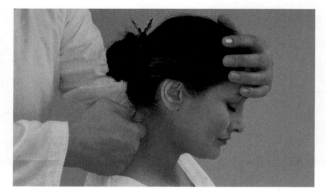

Fig. 10.82 *Step 10, Part 1*

Part 2
Thumb pushes – place your right thumb at the base of the neck (T1) on the spine and slide it forward, horizontally, across the side of the neck three times.

Repeat at the middle of the neck three times.

Repeat at the top of the neck three times.

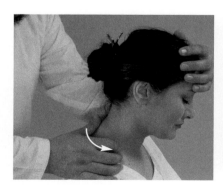 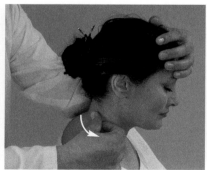 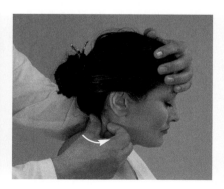

Fig. 10.83 *Step 10, Part 2*   **Fig. 10.84** *Part 2*   **Fig. 10.85** *Part 2*

Part 3

Finger pulls – still working with your left hand, place the side of the forefinger slightly in front of the base of the neck, with the thumb anchored at the spine, and pull the forefingers back towards the thumb three times.

Repeat at the middle of the neck three times.

Repeat at the base of the neck three times.

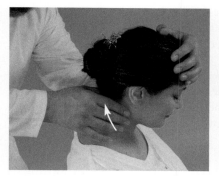

Fig. 10.86 *Step 10, Part 3*

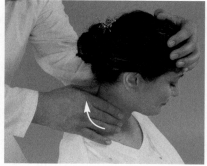

Fig. 10.87 *Part 3*

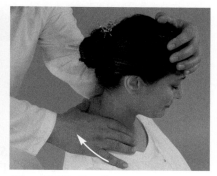

Fig. 10.88 *Part 3*

Part 4

Gentle neck stretches – place your left forearm on the client's left shoulder. Ask the client to take a deep breath in and then gently stretch three times when the client breathes out.

Step 11

Repeat steps 9 and 10 to the other side of the neck.

Step 12

Friction to the base of the skull – support the client's forehead with your hand, stand on the client's right side, and with all the fingers of the other hand, work your way up and down from behind the left ear to the spine. Repeat on the opposite side, three times.

Step 13

Heel rub under the occipital bone – with your right hand on the client's forehead, tilt the head slightly forward. Rub the base of the skull lightly and briskly with the heel of your left hand, from behind the left ear to the spine. Repeat on the opposite side, three times.

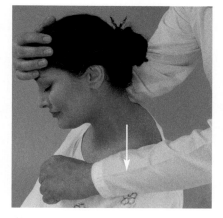

Fig. 10.89 *Part 4*

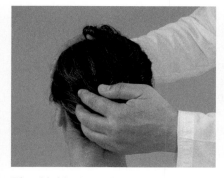

Fig. 10.90 *Step 12*

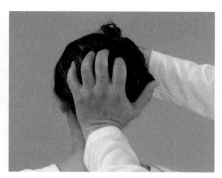

Fig. 10.91 *Step 13*

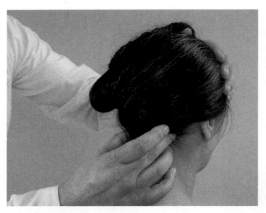

Fig. 10.92 *Step 14*

Step 14

Siramatrika and krikatika marma points – place one hand on the client's forehead, and with the thumb and middle finger of the other hand, gently rotate anti-clockwise and clockwise along the eight siramatrika marma points (a fingerwidth apart) along the length of the base of the skull from both ear bones, meeting at the centre of the occiput at the two krikatika marma points.

Benefits of stimulating the siramatrika marma points
- Loosens the muscles of the face and jaw
- Alleviates noises in the ears
- Assists the clearing of middle-ear congestion

Benefits of stimulating the krikatika marma points
- Unwinds the whole body via the spine reflexes
- Mitigates pain in the back of the head and neck tension
- May assist in improvement of hearing

Step 15

Effleurage the base of the client's skull and neck three times, by moving your left hand diagonally up and across the neck, and repeating with the right hand.

Cradle the head with both hands so the neck is straight and the face up, to calm and ground the energy.

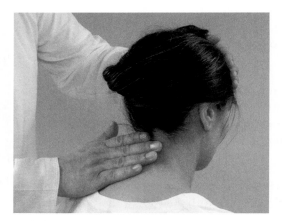

Fig. 10.93 *Step 15*

Benefits
- Loosens and tones the muscles of the neck
- Stimulates the thyroid gland which generates flow of fresh energy throughout the body
- Balances the electromagnetic energies in the right and left side of the brain. This reduces stress as it increases the brain's ability to deal with incoming information, bringing both the logical and intuitive responses together
- Aids the regulation of the thyroid gland

Scalp

Step 1

Part 1

Oil

Place a medium-size towel around the client's neck and tie a knot at the front of the neck.

Part 2

Standing at the side of the client, position the heel of your right hand in the dip of the client's nose, and stretch your palm and fingers towards the middle of the client's head. With your left hand measure two fingers' width from the end of your right hand's middle finger. Where your middle finger sits is the adipathi marma point. With your right hand, apply about 20 ml of warm sesame oil through a squeeze-top bottle.

> **REMEMBER**
> The adapathi marma point is one of the 108 therapeutic junction points on the head. It is where blood, vessels, nerves and lymphatics, as well as Vata, Pita and Kapa doshas, convene.

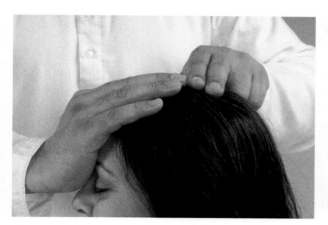

Fig. 10.94 *Step 1, Part 2*

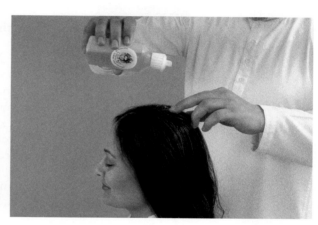

Fig. 10.95 *Step 1, Part 2*

Part 3

Neck flexion and extension (roll) – stand behind the client, place your hands on either side of her head and gently roll the head three times anti-clockwise and clockwise.

Spread your fingers and hold the head firmly so that it does not escape from your hands. In your rotation, attempt to touch the client's chin to the chest, the left ear to the left shoulder, comfortably lean the head towards the back, and the right ear to the right shoulder (as in step 1, part 1 of the neck technique) so as to evenly spread the oil.

Remember that as you have applied oil to the scalp, with the neck flexion and extension (roll) movement, you will need to make firm contact with the scalp so that you can stop the oil from running down.

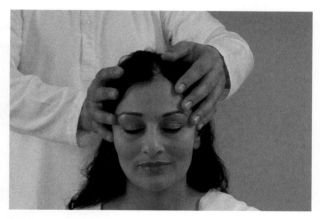

Fig. 10.96 *Part 3*

Step 2

Part 1

Rubbing – standing behind the client, support the right side of her head and use the ball of your left hand to carry out a light rubbing movement from the hairline to the occiput.

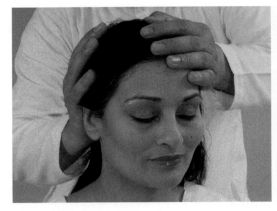

Fig. 10.97 *Step 2, Part 1*

Part 2

Alternate movements, i.e. left and right side of the client's scalp. Repeat three times on both sides of the client's scalp so that the oil does not escape.

Step 3

Finger friction – standing behind the client, support the right side of the head with your right hand. Use all of the fingers of your left hand to stimulate the left side of the client's scalp with zig-zag movements, from the hairline, over the head to the back of the skull. Apply sufficient pressure so that skin is moved back and forth on the skull bones.

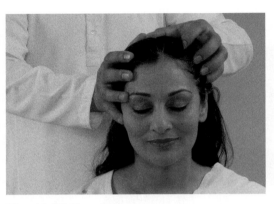

Fig. 10.98 *Step 3*

Alternate movements, i.e. left and right side of the client's scalp. Repeat three times on both sides of the client's scalp.

> **GOOD PRACTICE**
>
> Be sensitive to the individual. Thin people usually need less pressure and speed than heavier people with thick scalps to get the same result.

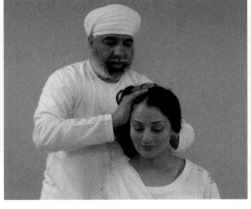

Fig. 10.99 *Step 4*

Step 4

Whole-hand friction – standing behind at one corner of the client, support the South West quarter of the head with your left hand, and with the right hand, apply firm rubbing movements to the North East quarter. Repeat to the other diagonal sides, i.e. NW to SE.

> **GOOD PRACTICE**
>
> Always support the side of the head you are not working on so the recipient does not have to brace her neck to hold it in position for you.

Step 5

Tug at hair – standing behind the client, slide your fingers underneath the client's hair. Take a section at a time, clench your fingers and make sure that the roots of the hair are grasped. Allow your right knuckles to rotate the scalp anti-clockwise and clockwise three times. Your left wrist will automatically follow the movement of the right wrist, like cycling where one foot will follow the other.

Start with East-West, followed by NE-SW, North-South, and NE-SW.

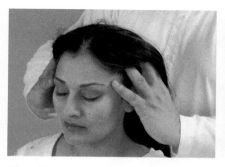

Fig. 10.100 *Step 5*

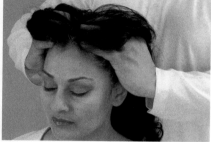

Fig. 10.101 *Step 5*

Step 6

Claw – standing behind the client, place your hands either over or under the client's hair so that the heels of your hands sit just under the ears. With your elbows apart, the heels of your hands should squeeze inward with medium pressure, lift the scalp from the skull, and release.

Start with East-West, followed by NE-SW, North-South, and NE-SW.

Step 7

Deep scalp friction – standing at the side of the client, massage with thumb and fingertips from hairline and occupit with deep slow movements to the whole of the scalp, meeting at the adipathi. Repeat three times.

Standing behind the client, repeat the above process starting above the ears and again finishing at the adipathi. Repeat three times.

Step 8

Effleurage – standing behind your client, run your fingertips through the hair from the hairline towards the back of the head (you may also use nails to comb through hair), covering the entire surface of the scalp.

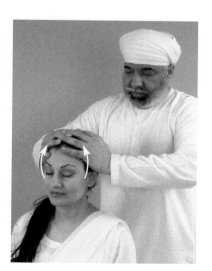

Fig. 10.102 *Step 6*

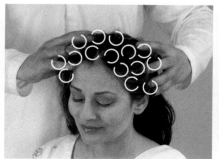

Fig. 10.103 *Step 7*

Fig. 10.104 *Step 8*

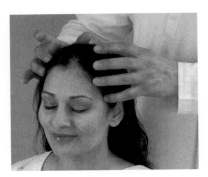

Fig. 10.105 *Step 9*

Step 9

Tapping – using the pads of your fingers, gently tap over the entire surface of the client's scalp, while moving around the client.

Step 10

Support the client's head with your right hand and use your left hand to work from the hairline towards the back of the head covering the left side of the scalp. Gently rotate the thumb and fingertips anti-clockwise and clockwise with gentle pressure. Re-anchor your fingers 1cm back towards the occiput after each rotation – the thumb stays along the centre line. This procedure is carried out once only, not three times.

Repeat on the right side of the client's scalp.

Step 11

Gentle effleurage and stroking to scalp (as in step 7).

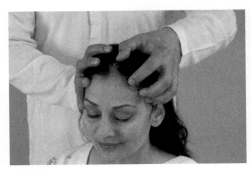

Fig. 10.106 *Step 10*

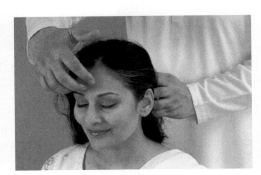

Fig. 10.107 *Step 11*

Step 12

Lay both hands on the client's head to finish, then wash your hands with anti-bacterial soap.

Benefits
- Facilitates the release of serotonin into the blood stream, which gives a sense of pleasure and satisfaction and elevates the mood
- Regulates hormone release by stimulating the pituitary and pineal glands
- Facilitates the reduction of high blood pressure
- Helps to relieve frontal tension headaches
- Relieves dizziness and ringing in the ears
- Increases the flow of cerebro-spinal fluid
- Helps in the relief of insomnia
- Helps to improve the memory
- Creates alertness
- Relieves neck tension
- Relieves tension headaches
- Improves mental clarity and ability to concentrate
- Helps in the balancing and regulating of sensory and motor centres in the brain

Facial massage

(Please see Chapter 11 for information on Ayurvedic Facial Rejuvenation Treatment.)

Step 1

Part 1

Cover the client's head with the towel placed around the client's neck, so that you do not get oil on your tunic top. Gently guide the client's head from the base of the neck to lean on your front. Roll up a separate towel and place between the client's neck and you for the client's maximum comfort.

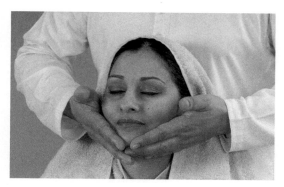

Fig. 10.108 *Step 1, Part 1*

GOOD PRACTICE

Roll up a towel and place it between you and the client's neck.

Part 2

Cover your palms with a light amount of warm sesame oil. Place your index finger at the shringatakani lower marma point, below the lower lip, and your thumb at the tip of the chin. With both of your hands firmly effleurage from under the chin and jaw, moving up in front of and above the ears, to finish behind the ears. Repeat three times.

Pay special attention to the area at the root of the tongue and the tonsils, as a lot of tension collects here. This is particularly so if the client feels awkward about voicing her thoughts and feelings.

The muscles of the jaw hold a lot of tight habit patterns, some of which cause considerable discomfort in the neck as well as the face. The jaw muscle is actually the strongest muscle in the group, so tension here can trap a lot of body energy. If it appears that there is a lot of jaw tension, ask the client to open her mouth as wide as possible. In your post-treatment advice encourage the client to repeat this exercise a few times a day. Reading aloud to oneself while holding a cork between the front teeth is another great technique to loosen the jaw.

REMEMBER
People who are stressed may suffer jaw tension.

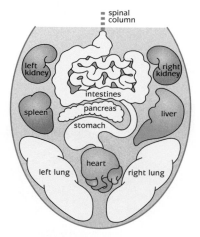

Fig. 10.108a *Tongue diagnosis*

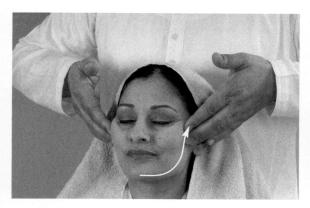

Fig. 10.109 *Step 1, Part 2*

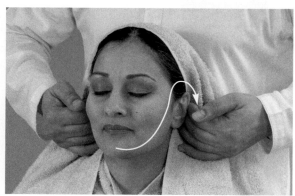

Fig. 10.110 *Step 1, Part 2*

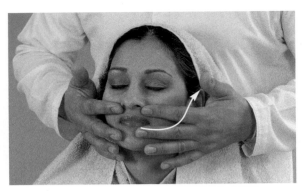

Fig. 10.111 *Step 2*

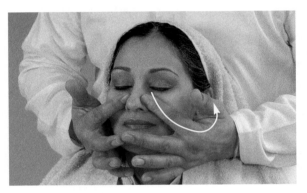

Fig. 10.112 *Step 2*

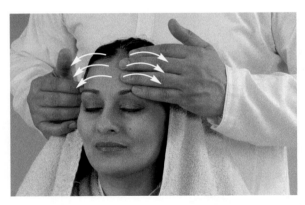

Fig. 10.113 *Step 3*

Step 2
Part 1
With the client's head still leaning against your body, place the tips of your index fingers at usta marma point, midway between the client's nose and the middle of the upper lip. Rotate this point anti-clockwise and clockwise three times. Then firmly effleurage across and underneath the cheeks by moving up in front and above the ears, to finish behind the ears. Repeat three times.

Give special attention along the jaw to the midpoint of the muscles that open and close the jaw. With your index fingers rotate anti-clockwise and clockwise three times.

Part 2
Place the tips of your index fingers at the nasa marma point, just above the flare of the client's nostrils. Rotate this point anti-clockwise and clockwise three times, then firmly effleurage across underneath the cheeks by moving up in front of and above the ears, to finish behind the ears. Repeat three times.

Part 3
Place the tips of your index fingers at the ganda marma point, on the either side of the client's nose, midway between the inner corner of the eyes and the nasa marma point. Rotate this point anti-clockwise and clockwise three times, then firmly effleurage across underneath the cheeks by moving up in front of and above the ears, to finish behind the client's ears. Repeat three times.

Step 3
With the client's head still leaning against your body, with smoothing strokes, starting from the midline of the client's forehead using both of your hands, effleurage across the forehead to finish behind the ears. Repeat three times.

Benefits
- Releases emotions
- Relieves temporomandibular joint (TMJ) syndrome
- Increases blood circulation to the face
- Brings a rosy, healthy glow to the cheeks
- Causes salivation, keeping the mouth moist
- Brings warmth and relaxation to the muscles
- Builds muscle tone helping to prevent lines and wrinkles
- Fills out the sunken tissues, softening the angles of the face
- Warm oil relaxes the muscles beneath the skin. It also 'feeds' the skin. Sesame oil penetrates the skin's outer layers
- Releases jaw tension, helping verbal expression and releasing grinding of the teeth

- Therapeutic movements bring focus back to the face and head, which is where the greater part of the massage takes place. It also helps the client to be still and focus their own energy once again.

Underlying causes of TMJ syndrome include:
- TMJ muscle tension
- TMJ muscle spasm
- Emotional stress
- Teeth grinding
- Dental bite misalignment
- Poorly fitted dentures
- Partial jaw dislocation
- Jaw injury
- Headaches
- Pain in the temples, neck, shoulders and back
- Diminished hearing
- Sinus problems

The source of the problem is actually constant jaw clenching or teeth grinding. Over a period of time, the muscles that control the temporomandibular joints (where the jaw joins the skull) develop nodules that produce the symptoms when aggravated.

Step 4

Part 1

With the client's head still leaning against your body, begin above the bridge of the client's nose (inner end of the eyebrow). Secure your index fingers on the top ridge of the eye socket and allow the pads of your thumbs, with firm pressure, to roll down from the client's hairline, to meet your index fingers. Repeat three times.

Part 2

Repeat as above the at client's mid-eyebrow. Repeat three times.

Part 3

Repeat as above, at the end of the client's eyebrow.

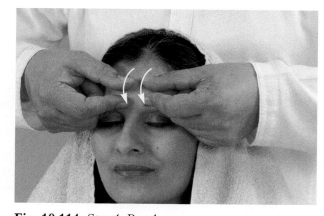

Fig. 10.114 *Step 4, Part 1*

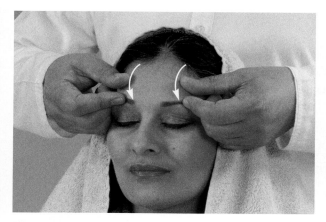

Fig. 10.115 *Part 2*

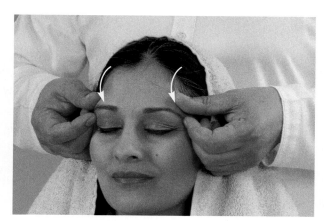

Fig. 10.116 *Part 3*

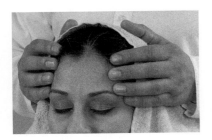

Fig. 10.117 *Step 4, Part 4*

Part 4
Emotional stress release

Rest the pads of your fingers on each corner of the client's forehead until you feel a pulse.

Emotions can be a primary factor in muscle imbalances and aggravate physical problems arising from other sources. Knowing how to take emotional stress out of the situation promotes recovery.

Emotional stress release (ESR) is a great technique to get the mind and feelings back in control. It permits the intellect to go to work finding positive alternatives with which to handle troublesome situations. ESR does not solve problems but it helps the client deal with stress more efficiently.

Use four fingers (as in the illustration) to touch the neuro-vascular holding points. Apply only enough pressure until the pulses in the frontal eminences synchronise. Ask the client to 'think back to the beginning of the incident and all the way through until you have come to the end or to the point where you are now with the incident. When you get to the end, flex your right hand.'

ESR works well in getting relief from nightmares, fears, frustrations and other problems that affect personal and professional efficiency and creativity.

Step 5
Part 1 and part 2 are done just once.

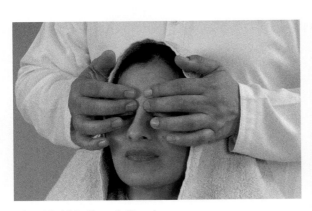

Fig. 10.118 *Step 5, Part 1*

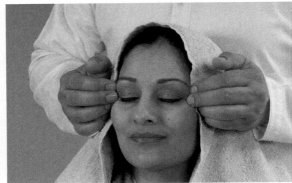

Fig. 10.119 *Step 5, Part 1*

Part 1
Eye orbit
With the client's head still leaning against you, situate the heels of your hands on the client's temple region. Place your index and middle fingertips at the agya chakra (third eye), between the client's eyebrows.

Gently press, rotate anti-clockwise and clockwise and in tiny steps move along the top ridge of the client's eye socket to the apanga marma points.

Do not pull on the client's skin but re-anchor the tiny steps with your thumbs.

Part 2
Now coil your fingers and place the back of your fingers on the client's cheeks. From the apanga marma point rotate anti-clockwise and clockwise with the edge of your thumb, along the bottom ridge of the eye socket, ending at the shringatakani upper marma points.

Again do not pull on the client's skin but re-anchor the tiny steps with your thumbs.

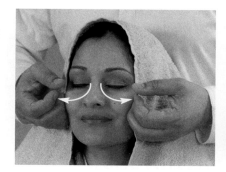

Fig. 10.120 *Step 5, Part 2*

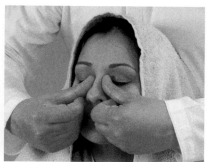

Fig. 10.121 *Step 5, Part 2*

Part 3
From the shringatakani upper marma points, drain the side channels of the client's nose by rotating the edge of your thumbs in very small circles to the nasa marma points at either side of the nose.

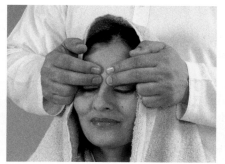

Fig. 10.122 *Part 3*

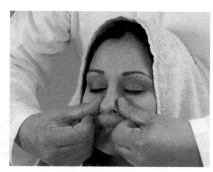

Fig. 10.123 *Part 3*

Part 4
Leave your index fingertips at the nasa marma points and drain sinuses by curving your forefingers under the cheekbones. Ask the client to take a deep breathe in and very gently pull up the zygomata, and then ask the client to breathe out and release the zygomata. Repeat twice. Always make sure that you deliver instructions to the client that are followed by your actions.

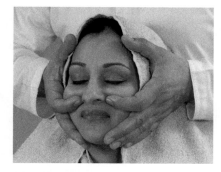

Fig. 10.124 *Part 4*

Benefits
- Assists in reducing hyperactivity
- Facilitates memory improvement
- Increases blood circulation to the brain
- Increases the power of concentration
- Assists in relieving tension headaches
- Relieves tired eyes and improves eyesight
- Helps to nourish and relax the nervous system
- Clears perceptions and brings peace to the mind
- Assists in the relief of asthma and bronchial congestion
- Builds muscle tone helping to prevent lines and wrinkles

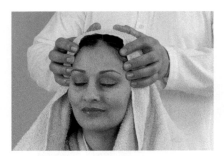

Fig. 10.125 *Step 6*

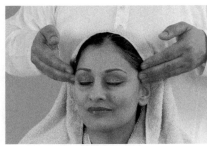

Fig. 10.126 *Step 6*

Step 6

With the client's head still leaning against you, use your fingers to create gentle circular anti-clockwise and clockwise friction movements to the client's temple region, around the shakha marma points. Clear the hair away from the ears.

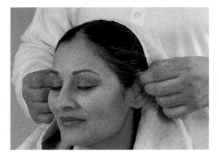

Fig. 10.127 *Step 7, Part 1*

Step 7

Part 1

With the client's head still leaning against you, hold the ear lobe between your thumb and index finger. With a rolling gentle squeezing motion, move along the outer edge of the ear to the point where the ear connects to the head, and work back down. Apply oil around the ear lobe and entrance to the ear canal. Gently pull the ear up.

Part 2

Work in a similar way along the middle ridge of the ear and apply oil. Gently pull the ear back towards you.

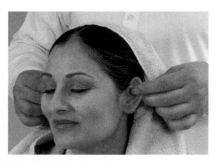

Fig. 10.128 *Part 2*

Part 3

Use the tip of your index fingers to rub the innermost part of the ear and apply oil. Gently pull the ear down.

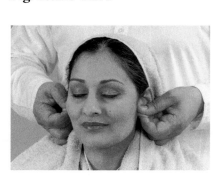

Fig. 10.129 *Part 3*

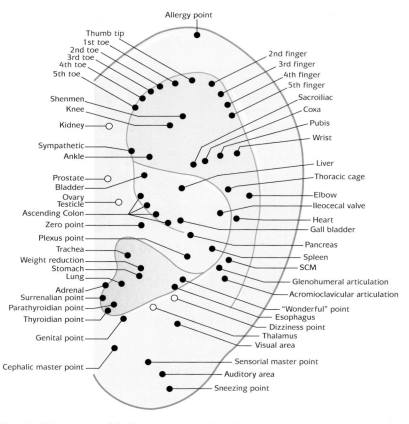

Fig. 10.129a *Parts of the body represented on the ear*

Benefits

- Relieves tension and can assist in correcting deformities of the spine
- Aids low back pain, improves stamina and energises kidneys
- Stimulates the central nervous system
- Facilitates improvement in circulation
- Helps to balance the Vata dosha
- Lowers high blood pressure
- Aids excretory functions

Step 8

Part 1

Gentle hand placing

With the client's head still leaning against you, rub your hands together until they are warm. Gently place hands so that palms cover the ears and forefingers rest on lthe ower part of the client's cheeks.

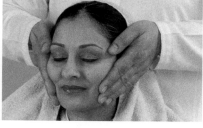

Fig. 10.130 *Step 8, Part 1*

Part 2

Place your hands so the tip of the middle fingers meet at the bridge of the client's nose covering the eyes.

Part 3

Place your hands on top of the client's head.

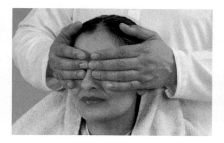

Fig. 10.131 *Part 2*

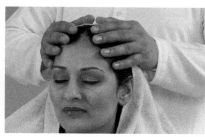

Fig. 10.132 *Part 3*

Step 9

Colours can have a huge effect on our mood, so use them to your advantage. Suggest that the client visualises the appropriate colour when you are working on their chakras.

Part 1

Rub your hands together until they are warm. Kneel at the side of the client, place one hand above the Sahasrar chakra (crown), while the other hand cups (without touching) the client's Mooladhar chakra (root). Visualise the colour red and take five deep breaths.

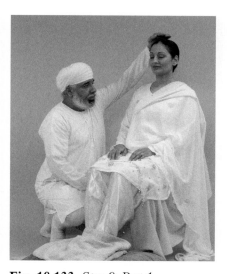

Fig. 10.133 *Step 9, Part 1*

Part 2
Maintain one hand above the Sahasrar chakra, while the other hand cups the client's Svadishthana chakra (sacral). Visualise the colour orange and take five deep breaths.

Part 3
Maintain one hand above the Sahasrar chakra, while the other hand cups the client's Manipur chakra (solar plexus). Visualise the colour lemon and take five deep breaths.

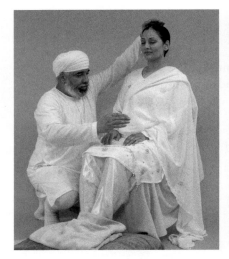

Fig. 10.134 *Part 2*

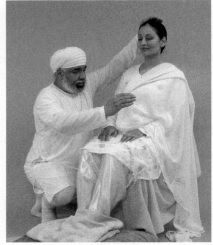

Fig. 10.135 *Part 3*

Part 4
Stand to the side of the client, maintain one hand above the Sahasrar chakra, while the other hand cups the client's Anahath chakra (heart). Visualise the colour emerald and take five deep breaths.

Part 5
Maintain one hand above the Sahasrar chakra, while the other hand cups the client's Vishudhi chakra (throat). Visualise the colour turquoise and take five deep breaths.

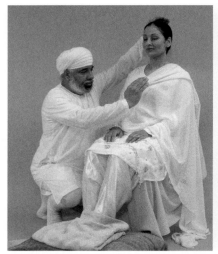

Fig. 10.136 *Part 4*

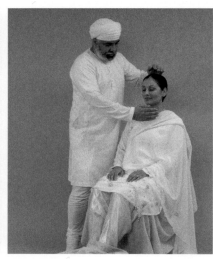

Fig. 10.137 *Part 5*

Part 6
Maintain one hand above the Sahasrar chakra, while the other hand cups the client's Agya chakra (third eye). Visualise the colour indigo and take five deep breaths.

Part 7
Hold both hands above the Sahasrar chakra. Visualise the colour white and take five deep breaths.

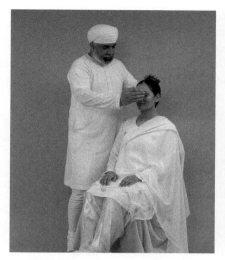

Fig. 10.138 *Part 6*

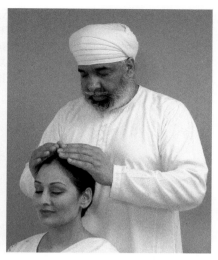

Fig. 10.139 *Part 7*

Benefits
- Opens the subconscious to be receptive to new inspirations
- Relieves congestion that causes bags to form under the eyes
- Relieves pressure around and in the eyeball, brightens the eyes
- Improves skin tone around the eye, relieving bags and darkness
- Makes the eyes water which releases emotions held in the eye sockets in a similar way to tears, also assists to relieve emotional tension
- Helps in the release of repressed emotions, especially anger, frustration and grief
- Massage of the temples helps to improve eyesight, creating a centred state of awareness
- Stimulates the delicate muscles around the temples to help lessen crow's feet
- Improves alertness which is useful in relieving dizziness or nausea and reviving someone from fainting
- Allows energy to flow through the eye socket, the nose, the mouth, the ears and the higher chakras, therefore allows a balance of the prana-chakra-nadi-marma matrix.

Table 10.01

	Chakras		Colour	Prana
7	Sahasrar	Crown	White	Working on the Sahasrar and Agya harmonises the Prana Vayu
6	Agya	Third eye	Indigo	
5	Vishudhi	Throat	Turquoise	Working on the Vishudhi harmonises the Udana Vayu
4	Anahath	Heart	Emerald	Anahath and Manipur calm both the Vyana and Prana Vayus
3	Manipur	Solar plexus	Lemon	
2	Svadishthana	Sacral	Orange	Svadishthana calms and harmonises the Samana Vayu
1	Mooladhar	Root	Red	Mooladhar harmonises the Apana Vayu

Step 10

Part 1

Sealing the treatment

While standing at the side of the client, rest one hand on the third eye. With the other hand grasp and pull back gently at the vertebrae up the neck.

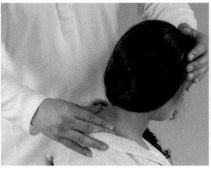

Fig. 10.140 *Step 10, Part 1*   **Fig. 10.141** *Step 10, Part 1*

Part 2

Effleurage each side of the upper back and across the shoulders three times each side. Support the client with your opposite hand on each occasion.

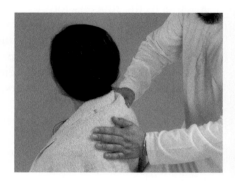

Fig. 10.142 *Part 2*

Part 3

Gently release your hands from the client's shoulders and spiral five circles, as if you are coming out of the client's aura. Shake your arms and hands to release stagnant prana, and embrace both hands to seal the treatment.

Part 4

Stand in front of the sitting client and gently ring a bell and inform her that the treatment has come to an end. Encourage her to move slowly when she feels ready. Take a few minutes to share this experience together and then offer a glass of water followed by post-treatment advice and book the next appointment. Return the client's shoes and remind them to collect their jewellery and belongings.

Progress Check

1. What is the purpose of Shiro-Abhyanga?
2. Why is preparation before the treatment so important?
3. State five things you can do to ensure client comfort throughout the treatment.

Key Terms

You need to know what these words mean. Go back through the chapter or check in the glossary to find out.

- Sahasar
- Marma points
- Agya
- Vishudhi
- Anahath
- Manipur
- Svadishthana
- Mooladhar

11 Ayurvedic Facial Rejuvenation Treatment

After working through this chapter you will be able to:

♦ Gain an understanding of Ayurvedic facial rejuvenation massage

♦ Learn more about nutrition for healthy eyes.

Understanding Ayurvedic facial rejuvenation

Modern lifestyle leads to poor health in many ways, but the use of simple and natural methods can significantly improve health and vitality. In Ayurveda, rejuvenating therapy optimises the circulation of nutrients to both body and mind, and is the holistic way to attain longevity as it is aimed at the preservation of health.

The human body, consisting of 50–100 million cells, when healthy is in harmony, is self-perpetuating and self-correcting, just as the universe is. The ancient Ayurveda text, *Charaka*, says, 'Man is the embodiment of the universe. Within man, there is as much diversity as in the world outside. Similarly, the outside world is as diverse as human beings themselves.' In other words, the basic premise of Ayurveda is that the entire cosmos or universe is part of one singular absolute.

REMEMBER
The basic premise of Ayurveda is that the entire cosmos or universe is part of one singular absolute.

Western medicine has, for the most part, focused its attention on putting substances (e.g. pharmaceuticals) into the body rather than taking unhealthy substances out. Therefore, an Indian Head Massage therapist might suggest that a client leaves out certain cosmetic products.

Over the years almost every culture has rediscovered the magic of touch for itself and formulated its own system of massaging and touching for health.

Today, massage, in its many forms is used to relieve stress, tension and emotional trauma; to heal physical damage to the muscles and skeletal supporting tissues; and simply as a pleasant thing to do as a form of communication.

Ayurvedic facial rejuvenation massage is based on the concept of the promotion of the free flow of blood and other nutrients to the facial area. It involves massage techniques that smooth away the impediments that tighten the facial muscles. The treatment targets the connective tissues beneath the facial skin and releases tension in them. It also relaxes the facial muscles. The combined action makes the face fresh, supple and lively. This treatment benefits not just the face but also the mind and body by bringing about mental tranquillity and metabolic vigour.

REMEMBER
Ayurvedic facial rejuvenation massage helps to reduce wrinkles on the face and bags under the eyes.

It helps to reduce wrinkles on the face and bags under the eyes by tightening the skin and jaw line. It is an extremely relaxing treatment which gently lifts your client's face to give it a more youthful, healthy look. There are 90 muscles in the face, which need to be used on a daily basis to keep them supple and toned. Both men and women can benefit from this treatment.

Through massage, the skin is gently manipulated so that it becomes more supple and elastic. Massage also helps to bring more nutrients and blood to the skin to nourish it and remove toxic build-up. As clients relax, the tension eases from their faces and they become happier, which in turn helps to reduce stress. For the best results, a course of treatment should be recommended.

For thousands of years Indian civilisations have enjoyed Ayurvedic facial rejuvenation treatments. It is a natural process conducted with natural ingredients for the ultimate natural face-lift. It is a better and more economical holistic method then having staples behind one's ears. The intricate massage for all the systems of the body is supported by the activation of the chakras, nadis, marma points and flow of the prana.

The introduction of Ayurveda into the modern beauty/aesthetics environment is like going 'back to the future'. Ancient ingredients and age-old procedures are racing towards the cutting edge of today's holistic beauty care. Therapists are aware that people today are coming to demand total natural bodycare. There is increasing interest in treatments that work not only to beautify the skin but also to nurture and relax the mind, body and spirit. Ayurveda is a leader in this 'new age' of self-care consciousness.

More and more experienced holistic aesthetician/beauty/complementary therapists acknowledge that natural cosmetics are more healthy and effective than their synthetic counterparts. Whether you make cosmetics at home or purchase them from a commercial source, test them on a small area of skin before you spread them all over your client's face. When working directly on the face, use cold-pressed, preservative-free vegetable oil or combinations of oils. Remember that just because the ingredients are pure and natural does not make them hypoallergenic. Ayurvedic skincare products are not tested on animals.

Tension gathers in the face causing the forehead, eye, jaw and mouth regions to tighten, which may result in headaches and eyestrain. Toothache is probably the most excruciating pain that we have all encountered at some stage in our lives. The intensity of local nerves in the face can, at times, be unbearable. Tension in the temple region constricts the flow of blood and can not only lead to headaches and eyestrain, but also to the hair turning grey around the temples as the hair roots are starved of nutrients.

The Vata face

The rejuvenating therapy addresses ageing, dryness, dehydration and stressed and tired skin by using a blend of herbal masks and essential oils. The skin is cleansed and toned with three types of rejuvenating massages, including marma therapy for scalp, neck and shoulders.

The Pita face

This purifying therapy treats toxicity, redness and sensitivity. The skin is purged using cooling and cleansing herbal formulas, to clean, tone and detoxify. This treatment is especially good for psoriasis, eczema, rosacea, acne and hypersensitivity.

The Kapa face

This deluxe therapy addresses the symptoms of both Vata and Pita faces. This customised experience is for combination skin; the face is cleansed, toned, steamed, stimulated, calmed, cooled, purified and rejuvenated.

Facial study

Fig. 11.01 *The Kapa face*

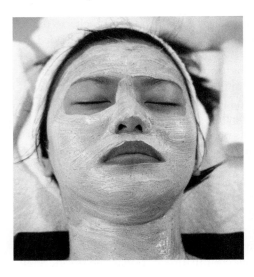

The face is the autobiography of life. It is exciting beyond words to look into a person's face with complete understanding and to recognise their atma and personality for what they truly are:

- The forehead indicates your frame of mind through which you perceive the world.
- Each individual feature or part speaks a unique language of its own.
- Structure indicates the potential for performance.
- The cheeks, lips and jaw all express who you really are.
- The eyes are a point of view while the nose 'knows' your personality.
- The issues are in the tissues.

The hypothesis is that the body's cells need essential minerals or tissue salts in order for our bodies to function efficiently. This means if supplies of these minerals run low, the body draws from its own resources. If a plant is unwell it turns several different colours before it finally goes black, because it is lacking certain vital minerals essential for survival. Our bodies react to mineral deficiencies in similar ways.

A qualified therapist looks for markings, facial colour and skin texture, which indicate where there might be mineral deficiencies. Horizontal lines that manifest around the client's forehead might indicate liver problems, while puffy eyes may suggest a blocked colon.

GOOD PRACTICE

A therapist will observe markings on the skin, its texture and also facial colour, which may indicate health problems.

Once an observation has been made, the therapist may recommend a tailor-made detox diet to suit the client. A typical detox regime may include Nasya, Pradhamana Nasya, Karna Purana, Netra Basti and dietary adjustment, depending on the client's dosha.

The maintenance plan has been designed to carefully balance the minerals, which affect our metabolic rate. An over-indulgence of certain foods could give you too many minerals of one kind – or not enough of another. This in turn affects how fast our body burns up fat and has an impact on our energy levels.

Massage to the face stimulates and improves scalp circulation and improves the strength, texture and growth of hair. It soothes and rebalances energy flow, creating a feeling of calm and wellbeing. Para-nasal sinus drainage movements enhance the holistic approach to Ayurvedic facial rejuvenation massage.

Healing hands also produce psychological benefits, balancing the higher chakra matrix and principally addressing the Agya chakra. The two physical eyes see the past and the present, while the third eye reveals the insight of the future. By releasing stagnant energy, it helps the body to work in a more harmonious manner as it works on the facial marma points.

People have always been fascinated with faces and their changing moods and expressions. It is not surprising that physiognomy – the ancient oriental art of reading someone's character from their outward appearance – came into being. King Solomon remarked that the heart of a man is open to the eyes of a wise man.

Benefits
The benefits include the following:

- Skin texture becomes softer
- Bagginess and puffiness are reduced
- Enhances nourishment and cleansing of tissues
- No expensive cosmetics that claim to offer the elixir of youth in a bottle
- The pores will be cleared of debris and the skin will feel wonderfully soft
- Extremely beneficial to eyes: improves vision, strengthens muscles and tissue surrounding the eyes
- Melts away facial tension and bodily stress, smoothing wrinkles and bringing gentleness to the expression
- No nip and tuck – Ayurvedic facial rejuvenation treatment means that you do not need cosmetic surgery to look younger
- The antidote to premature ageing is rasyana cikitsa, or anti-ageing therapy. This maintains good tone and elasticity to all skin layers, which helps to hold youthful contours, reversing the ageing process. The rate of ageing is the comparison of a person's actual chronological age with their apparent age. If one appears to be younger than one's chronological age, this is a sign of positive health, and the converse holds true. Parameters such as long- and short-term memory, skin texture and lustre, gait, quality of the hair and daily activities are the measures to take into consideration.

The massage sequences are part of a complex complete treatment, which includes:

1. Cleansing
2. Oleation massage
3. Herbal steam or compress
4. Gentle scrub
5. Cleansing mask/facial pack
6. Toning
7. Moisturising
8. Hydrating.

This chapter is designed to raise your awareness of the nature of Ayurvedic facial rejuvenation massage. It does not detail the above eight sequences, as it is assumed that the therapist will have gained sufficient knowledge to employ the Amrit (nectar) face and neck mask – a starter course of which may be given on its own, with excellent results.

Amrit (nectar) face and neck mask
Ayurvedic facial rejuvenation starts with a face-softening mask.

Preparation
(Generally suitable for most types of skin)

Ingredients required:

- One tablespoon of besan gram (100% pure ground chana dal) flour. Still used on the Indian sub-continent as a gentle body cleanser
- One tablespoon of natural yoghurt. It smooths, moisturises, tightens and tones the skin. If possible always use organic products which are free from additives
- Half a level teaspoon of turmeric powder. Turmeric has antiseptic qualities, which cleanses the skin. Still traditionally used to beautify a bride before her wedding day
- Half a teaspoon of fresh lemon juice.

Method
Method of application:

1. Mix the flour, yoghurt, turmeric and lemon juice into a soft paste.
2. Apply to the face and neck for 15 minutes and wash off with warm water using a soft flannel.
3. After application, the pores will be cleared of debris and the skin will feel wonderfully soft.

> **REMEMBER**
> As this mask does not contain any preservatives, make just enough for one application and disregard the rest.

Holistic beauty/aesthetics transforms the skin. It makes the face look immediately younger, the skin tighter and rejuvenated, and eliminates the signs of ageing by accelerating the synthesis of cellular regeneration, while hydrating and firming. For centuries Indian and Oriental women have received such unique holistic anti-ageing treatments that encourage the natural ability of the skin to heal itself.

Ayurvedic facial rejuvenation is a natural programme to learn, to further your studies from Shiro-Abhyanga, and add another string to your bow. However, you require the underpinning knowledge of the Indian Head

Massage syllabus before you can truly be trained in Ayurvedic facial rejuvenation.

Although it is wonderful to receive an Ayurvedic facial rejuvenation massage, to date there are very few trained in this holistic therapy in the western world. For those interested in certified training, please refer to the source appendix (p. 248) for training providers.

please refer to the source appendix (p. 248) for training providers.

Nutrition for healthy eyes

Twenty/twenty vision is mark of just how well a person can see. If you can see a 19mm letter at a distance of 6 metres (20 feet) then you have 20/20 vision.

Wearing contact lenses or glasses does nothing to fundamentally fix impairments in your vision; instead the use of such aids improves your vision only for those times you are wearing them. Originally, however, contact lenses were actually designed to correct the shape of your eyeballs: first you were given one set of lenses to wear for about three days, then a weaker set for another three days, and so on, until your eyes got better. Somewhere along the way, the notion of actually correcting someone's sight was forgotten.

What you eat has an influence on how well your body functions, and affects your eyes as well. Everything that is good for you in general is also good for your vision. The following is a list of supplements that are known to have an effect on your vision.

> **REMEMBER**
> It is important not to self supplement but to see a nutritionist/dietician to advise on the correct vitamins and mineral supplements for each individual.

Eye anatomy	Nutritional element
Sclera (the white of the eyeball)	Calcium Calcium phosphate, calcium carbonate
Conjunctiva (the covering of the sclera)	Vitamin B2 – Riboflavin Vitamin B12 – Cyanocobalamin and folic acid
Cornea	Vitamin A – Retinol
Lens	Vitamin C – Ascorbic Acid Vitamin E – dl-Alpha Tocopherol Acetate Vitamin B2 – Riboflavin
Ciliary muscle	Chromium – Chromium Chloride
Retina	Vitamin A – Retinol Zinc – Zinc Sulphate and other minerals
Macula (the area around the fova)	Vitamin B complex Xanthophylls – Lutein/Zeaxanthin
Macula degeneration	Selenium, Zinc, Taurene, Vitamin E
Eye fatigue, night-vision	Bilberry extract – Anthocyanosides
Circulation	Grape seed extract – Proanthocyanidins

Table 11.01 *Nutritional element chart for the eyes*

Smile

Do you have lines on your face? What kind of lines are they? The predominant mood of your life is shown by the wrinkles on your face. They can be frown lines or they can be smile lines. Crow's feet are the sign of years of smiles. Did you know that a smile saves energy? It uses twelve muscles to frown, but only four to smile. It is said that, if you go to bed with a slight smile on your face, you will relax more easily into a refreshing sleep. Everyone smiles in the same language.

Try deliberately smiling to someone who looks despondent – a smile can be passed on. Imagine visiting a doctor who did not smile, or trying to talk to a shop assistant who did not smile. Somehow it spoils a two-way communication and takes away confidence.

A smile can unwind many tense situations. There may be a very real problem, but a smile is an invitation to talk about it more easily. Children always seem to be doing something wrong, but a big smile first tells them you love them, even though you may not love their naughty ways. A gentle smile to someone ill or old will lift the heart more than words can say, particularly when combined with an unhurried loving touch. Smiles will heal, but frowns can fracture.

So smile a little more often and respond positively to others. Develop a sense of fun and an ability to laugh at yourself. Avoid sameness and be a little daring (or a lot). Do something for others without hope of a reward.

Progress Check

1. What are the benefits of Ayurvedic facial rejuvenation?
2. What is the difference between Vata, Pita and Kapa facial treatments?
3. What type of indicators on the face would suggest health-related problems?
4. State four ingredients found in the facial products.

Key Terms

You need to know what these words mean. Go back through the chapter or check in the glossary to find out.

- Rejuvenation
- Hypoallergenic
- Detox
- Physiognomy
- Amrit
- Nutritionist

Post-treatment Advice

After working through this chapter you will be able to:

- Provide individual post-treatment advice
- Learn about the importance of food and its effects on the body.

You are what you eat

Ayurveda advocates that food is the first medicine – you are what you eat. A holistic lifestyle develops our pure inner nature and diet plays an important part in this process. The human body needs food containing carbohydrates, fats, fibre, minerals, proteins and vitamins for two purposes – as fuel for energy and as raw material to repair itself.

A vegetarian diet has very low cholesterol levels and gives rise to fewer heart problems. A vegetarian is also less likely to suffer from arthritis, constipation, food poisoning, gallstones, high blood pressure or obesity, and is likely to eat greater quantities of nutritious fruit and vegetables than a meat eater might.

A holistic lifestyle develops our pure inner nature, and diet plays an important part in this process. The vedic scriptures divide food into three types:

1. Satvic, or pure diet, brings purity and calmness to the mind.
2. Rajasic, or stimulating diet, destroys the mind and body balance that is essential for happiness.
3. Tamasic, or impure and putrid foods, over-stimulate the mind and cause mental stress.

The Ayurvedic diet is based on pure, satvic foods, and advocates a vegetarian diet.

Pure foods calm the mind and sharpen the senses. People's food preferences reflect their level of mental purity and alter as they develop spirituality.

Include the six basic tastes in your diet on a daily basis, and if possible at every meal. The tastes also have their own influence on the subtle inner balance of the physiology.

1. Astringent – beans, lentils, apples, rhubarb, lettuce, unripe bananas
2. Bitter – green leafy vegetables, spinach, courgettes and turmeric
3. Pungent – spicy foods, chillies, watercress, garlic, onion, cumin
4. Salty – sea salt, olives, food with added salt
5. Sour – yoghurt, lemons, cheese and vinegar
6. Sweet – starchy vegetables, grains, milk, pasta, sweet fruits

> **REMEMBER**
> The human body needs food containing carbohydrates, fats, fibre, minerals, proteins and vitamins for two purposes – as fuel for energy and raw material to repair itself.

> **REMEMBER**
> Pure foods calm the mind and sharpen the senses.

Table 12.01 *Ayurvedic diet: Satvic*

'The foods which increase life, purity, strength, health, joy and cheerfulness, which are savoury and oleaginous, substantial and agreeable, are dear to the satvic people.'

–Vedas

A satvic diet is a karma-free diet, as it is soothing and nourishing to the body. It promotes cheerfulness, serenity and mental clarity. It helps to maintain mental poise and nervous equilibrium throughout the day.

It is easily digested and supplies maximum energy, increasing vitality, strength and endurance, and will help to eliminate fatigue.

Satvic foods:

Fresh and dried fruits, pure fruit juices, raw or lightly cooked vegetables, salads, grains, legumes, nuts, seeds, wholemeal breads, honey, fresh herbs, herbal teas, milk, butter, yoghurt, wholemeal bread, wholemeal pasta, beans, pulses etc.

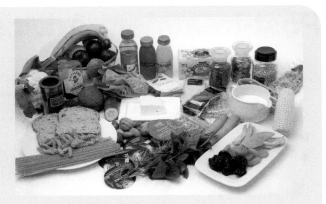

Fig. 12.01 *Satric foods*

These category foods are pure, wholesome and naturally delicious, without preservatives or artificial flavourings.

Table 12.02 *Ayurvedic diet: Rajasic*

'The foods that are bitter, sour, saline, excessively hot, pungent, dry and burning, are linked by the Rajasic and are productive of pain, grief and disease.'

–Vedas

Rajasic foods arouse animal passions, bring a restless state of mind and make the person overactive. These foods over-stimulate the body and cause physical stress and encourage circulatory and nervous disorders.

Rajasic foods:

Coffee, tea, tobacco, heavily spiced and salted foods, onions, garlic, chillies, radish, peppers, convenience snacks, refined sugar, soft drinks and chocolate.

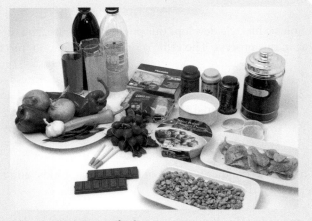

Fig. 12.02 *Rajasic foods*

Vegetables – asparagus, broccoli, brussels sprouts, cabbage, carrots, cauliflower, celery, courgettes, kale, leeks, lettuce, okra, onion, parsley, peas, potatoes, radish, spinach, spring greens, sweet peppers, sweet potatoes, cooked tomatoes, turnips, parsnips, watercress.

Fruits – apples, apricots, avocado, bananas, berries, blackcurrants, cherries, figs, grapefruit, grapes, kiwi, mangoes, melon, nectarines, papaya, peaches, pears, pineapple, plums, tangerines, watermelon.

Proteins – chickpeas, hummus, lentils, mung beans, soya beans, tofu.

Table 12.03 *Ayurvedic diet: Tamasic*

Tamasic

'That food which is stale, tasteless, putrid, rotten and impure, is the food liked by the Tamasic.'

–Vedas

Tamasic substances produce feelings of heaviness and lethargy. Foods that have been fermented, burned, fried, barbecued or re-heated many times, as well as stale products or those containing preservatives.

Overeating is tamasic. A tamasic diet benefits neither body nor mind. It makes a person dull and lazy, lacking in high ideals, purpose and motivation. Such individuals tend to suffer from chronic ailments and depression.

Tamasic foods:

Meat, fish, prawns, eggs, alcohol, recreational drugs, pickles, fried/grilled/barbecued foods.

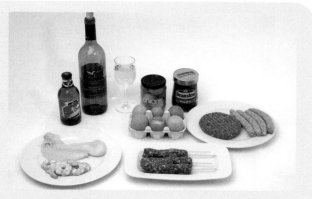

Fig. 12.03 *Tamasic foods*

Grains – barley, basmati rice, brown rice, buckwheat, millet, oats, pasta, wheatgerm, wholegrain breakfast cereals, wholemeal bread.

Herbs – aniseed, basil, black pepper, cayenne, chervil, chives, coriander, cumin, fennel, ginger, garlic, lemon, mint, oregano, parley, rosemary, sage, thyme, turmeric.

Nuts/Oils – almonds, brazil nuts, cashews, extra virgin olive oil, flaxseeds and oil, pumpkin seeds, sesame seeds, sunflower seeds (paste and oil), walnuts.

Eat to live, don't live to eat

Would you put your dinner on a dirty plate, with dried-on gravy from yesterday, and all the lumps and bits of previous meals still there? The thought is repugnant, but that is what most of us do with our bodies every day.

New food goes down on top of half-digested pieces of the previous snack, or on leftovers from breakfast that the stomach did not have time to deal with.

The alimentary canal through which our food passes is coated with deposits and so there is little active body surface available to assist the food as it moves along. The arteries can therefore become blocked with deposits of waxy cholesterol.

The cells are drowning in excess fluid or live in a permanent, stagnant, marshy swamp which does not allow them to get enough oxygen to function or be fed properly. To complete the picture, the main drain is blocked with constipation. The bacteria and toxins there thrive and multiply. To make things worse, if the rubbish cannot find its way out, it is partly reabsorbed into the body and infiltrates the tissues. All this provides the perfect conditions for illness and disease to develop.

Because the body fights quietly for a long time, we do not realise what is happening. Then the symptoms begin to appear – allergies, pains, infections, coughs and colds, sore throats, increased weight, diabetes, heart disease, the pains of arthritis, gall stones and other diseases have all been attributed to our way of eating. We are slowly killing ourselves. But it tastes nice while we do it, and we enjoy it!

A Russian minister of health in November 1996 said on ABC Television, 'Maybe we should be telling people their health is in their own hands. Doctors only deal with the consequences.'

There is no excuse for undermining the health of the human body, the most wondrous creation of the source, perfect in every detail.

Over-fed, undernourished

Ayurveda provides the perfect knowledge base for excellent detox remedies and treatments. Here are the basic top Ayurvedic detox tips for your health and rejuvenation. Many 'modern' detoxification methods use radical procedures to rid the body of waste products. Such treatments can disturb the delicate balance of mind and body, quite apart from the dangers of the body becoming inundated with the dissolved waste products and the purificatory system being overloaded. Pills, drinks and stick-on patches will not rid them of toxins.

Have a liquid diet – fruit and/or vegetable juices – for one day in every two weeks. Forty (holy) days is a significant figure in most religions and the theme is addressed not just for physical health, but benefits the mind as well. Mind and body detox periods based on religious institutions suggest a mandatory 40–day fast at least once a year. This is observed in Hinduism, as well as other Sanatan Dharam-based religions including Buddhism, Jainism and Sikhism. The same concept is duplicated by the three Middle Eastern sister religions. In Christianity, Ash Wednesday marks the start of Lent, when Christians traditionally give up eating and drinking something they like for 40 days, and Islam's Ramadan is a tradition where food is not eaten during daylight hours for 40 days.

> **REMEMBER**
> When beginning a detox diet you may feel worse before you feel better.

When you first start to change your diet and begin to eat many more raw foods, you may be puzzled to find that you feel more unwell. This is discouraging, but in actual fact is a natural reaction.

Over the years, particularly if the staple articles of diet have included 'junk food', then the chances are that some of the bowel is coated with residues that are now being shifted by the effect of raw fruits and juices. When these accretions are loosened, toxins come into the bloodstream, so it is understandable that we will not feel completely well.

This cleansing process can affect several parts of the body. There is a tendency to feel like the 'flu or a cold is coming on. The nose may run and fill with mucus. There is a strong likelihood of headaches and pains in joints. If the rubbish is coming out through the skin, your body may smell sour or you may develop spots. It is possible that it may come out directly from the bowel. It could appear like diarrhoea or your stools could be very loose, and perhaps be smelly. Every time you experience this, it means that the toxins of years are coming away.

If you have lived quite carefully, then this period may not last more than a few days, but could be longer if your lifestyle has been poor for many years. It is possible that there could be further healing crises but with each episode they will be shorter lasting.

It is worth being aware of this, as it can be upsetting if you think you have changed your lifestyle to something better and then become ill. Do not let anyone discourage you. Do not go back on what you are doing, thinking that fresh foods do not agree with you, or you will have to start all over again.

How can you survive this period? Because your body is working very hard to be healed and clean, it would be wise not to undertake any heavy work. Rest is the key and also plenty of water – up to four litres a day. Sometimes it can be helpful to have juice as well, particularly fresh carrots. The body has to deal with chemicals in foods through the liver, and it can become very overworked.

It will not be long before you find that you will suddenly have an exciting surge of energy and optimism, and realise that it has all been worthwhile.

Foods also affect the mind, emotions and the spiritual life. Ayurvedic doctrine suggests that of food or drink, the first third is gross and goes towards excrement and urine, the middle third goes to flesh and blood, while the most subtle third goes to the mind and atma.

> **REMEMBER**
> Food also affects the mind, emotions and the spiritual life.

The British Parliament Health Select Committee (HSC) warns 'this will be the first generation where children die before their parents'. Heart disease, strokes, some cancers and diabetes are classed as direct effects of obesity and excess weight. The HSC adds: 'People are now eating too much for the amount of physical activity they do." The modern-day culture of being 'over-fed but undernourished' is having a great impact on the eating habits of North America and Europe.

Post-treatment advice

Post-treatment advice is the therapist's prescription to the client. It forms the basis of recording the client's progress, and on each visit the client's prescription changes. For example, the therapist does not continue to offer the same advice time and time again. A client who may not drink any water may be encouraged to start by drinking one glass a day, and slowly build up the intake to a litre in one day over subsequent visits to the therapist. Always gain feedback from the client to establish immediate impressions and feelings and record them.

> **REMEMBER**
> Practise what you preach, by adopting a more potent change not only in your own lifestyle, but more importantly in your mind style.

Attempt to encourage your clients to sustain the post-treatment advice for at least 24 hours. Inevitably, over a course of treatment, as your Indian Head Massage treatments build up the client's immune system, their lifestyle will improve. It is for this reason that you need to practise what you preach, by adopting a more potent change not only in your own lifestyle, but more importantly in your mind style.

Diet

Drink plenty of water following the treatment – it helps to flush out toxins that have been released. Start by drinking a glass of water at room temperature, left overnight by your bedside. Follow a regime of drinking half a glass of still water with a slice of fresh ginger or lemon, at room temperature, on the hour, every hour, until evening. The important thing here is the frequency rather than the quantity. The bloodstream can only accommodate a certain amount of water and any excess may lead to erosion of minerals from the body. The purer the water you drink, the cleaner your body.

There are an astonishing number of chemicals in circulation, of which many have been banned for safety reasons but still linger in our water supply. The effect can range from hormone disorder to reproductive problems. Avoid ice-cold drinks as they dampen down the digestive processes.

Water is like engine oil, ensuring everything flows effortlessly and transporting energy-dense nutrients around the body. Dehydration also causes fatigue – with less fluid the heart has to work harder to pump blood.

Regular drinking of warm water balances both vata and kapa doshas, strengthens the digestive power, and helps to eliminate ama (metabolic waste products).

Cut down on tea, coffee and cola drinks, which should be avoided as they contain caffeine, a stimulant that will not help the client to relax. Stick to water, herbal teas and fresh juices.

Caffeine affects receptors in the brain, blocking the natural chemical adenosine. The knock-on effect is that your heart is stimulated and your body releases adrenaline. Caffeine can also irritate the bowel and aggravate symptoms of irritable bowel syndrome.

Avoid alcoholic beverages. Our lives have their difficulties, which worry us constantly as we move through life. Healthy choices help us to cope with whatever life puts in our way without having to resort to synthetic escapes such as alcohol. Alcohol will not provide a solution but, in fact, adds to the burdens.

If you normally drink three pints of lager a day, stopping would cut out 5,000 calories a week, and could help you shed a stone. You would also reduce the risk of heart attack or stroke by lowering unhealthy fats called triglycerides.

Exclude meat and fish and eat a light diet. If the body is using energy to digest a heavy meal it is not putting its energy into healing. Advise clients to eat raw foods such as vegetables and fruits for their vitality and cleansing effect. Consider the effects of non-organic foods, e.g. wheat, sugar, coffee, dairy products.

Most fast food contains too much salt, sugar, fat, preservatives and colourings, which can make you fat, slow your digestion, and lower your energy levels. Eliminate animal fats, meat, shellfish, saturated fats, margarine, lard, refined oils and fried foods.

Eat only when genuinely hungry and when your last meal is fully digested (about three to six hours after a main meal). Avoid eating between meals. Instead drink warm water, or if necessary eat ripe, sweet fruit.

Eat in a quiet and relaxed atmosphere. While eating you should not read, work or watch television. Always sit down to eat. Turning off the television can bring huge health benefits – it forces families to adopt a healthier lifestyle. A recent study found children who watch for two hours or more a day are more likely to smoke, be overweight and have high cholesterol.

Do not over-eat. After eating, the stomach should be only up to three-quarters full. Sit quietly for five to ten minutes at the end of each meal. Try to be regular in your meal times. Eat at the same times each day.

Your food should be freshly prepared; it should be wholesome and should taste good. Avoid reheated or stale food. Only eat unprocessed whole fresh foods. Look at your plate and ask yourself how close your food is to nature! Avoid preservatives, colourings and flavour enhancers in your food. Always read labels.

You don't get any nutritional benefits from sweets, and sucking on them all day is appalling for your teeth and puts you at real risk of tooth decay. Shunning sugar will reduce your waistline and your risk of diabetes. Too much sugar in your diet causes sugars to build up in your blood. This releases insulin, which mops up excess sugar and stores it as fat.

Cutting down your salt intake will lower your blood pressure, and with it your risk of stroke.

Hair and scalp care

Good hair and scalp care is important. Regular brushing distributes natural oils (sebum) and stimulates blood to the scalp. Use gentle, natural hair-care products that do not strip the hair's natural oils. Consider the effects of chemicals that you install for hair and scalp care, i.e. shampoos, conditioners, hair colours, sprays and gels, etc.

We naturally lose between 50 and 100 strands of hair every day. It takes a couple of weeks for hair to re-grow from the same follicle. The average scalp has about 100,000 hairs. Scalp hair grows at a rate of about 1 cm (just under half an inch) a month. Brushing your hair with 100 strokes every day can damage the hair shaft, and break hair, so it is better to massage the scalp.

Like the rest of the body, hair is closely related to prana. This is why, like Samson, none of India's Rishis (seers) ever cut their hair. They allowed it to grow as long as it liked and to break off when it chose to do so. Because healthy hair rarely grows on an unhealthy body, the hair and its lustre are important indicators of overall tissue health.

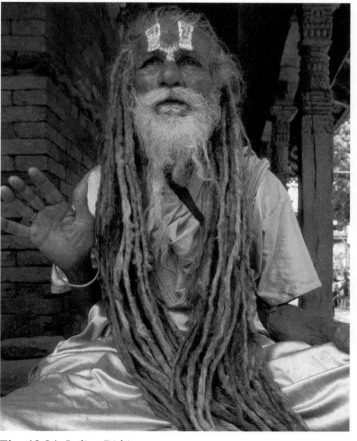

Fig. 12.04 *Indian Rishi*

Your hair is the barometer of your inner health. Healthy hair depends on a healthy diet. No amount of conditioners, colours, perming or styling aids can transform hair that has been starved of essential nutrients. The worst thing you can do for your hair is live on a diet of refined carbohydrates, processed foods, fizzy drinks, sugar, saturated and hydrogenated fats, caffeine, cigarettes and chocolate.

Essential nutrients for the hair

Protein – hair follicles have extremely high requirements for essential amino acids. Natural sources include tofu, pulses, grains, nuts, seeds and organic dairy products.

Iron – important for hair growth, a lack of it can result in thinning hair. Natural sources include dark green leafy vegetables, tofu and pulses.

Vitamin C – needed for healthy body tissue, including hair. It also helps the body to absorb iron. Natural sources include broccoli, spinach, cabbage, cauliflower, kiwi fruit, strawberries, oranges and grapefruit.

Vitamin E – this is needed to help develop and maintain strong cells. Vitamin E is also a powerful antioxidant. Natural sources include avocados, blackberries, mangoes, tomatoes, organic wholegrain cereal and vegetable oils.

Vitamin B complex – important for healthy hair. Natural sources include brown rice, wholegrain cereals, wheatgerm, green vegetables and organic dairy products.

Zinc – helps prevent dandruff. Natural sources include wholegrain breads and brown rice.

Excessive hair loss or thinning, known as alopecia, is becoming more and more widespread. Hair loss may be hereditary or may be caused by local bacterial, viral or fungal infections, or the chemicals we pour onto our scalps. Emotional stress, causing tension in the scalp, can also lead to abnormal hair loss, and many trichologists recommend relaxation techniques and Indian Head (scalp) Massage to treat these problems successfully.

Appearance

Deodorants – some sources suggested that since a woman is eight times more likely to develop breast cancer in the area closest to her underarm, there may be a link with the use of chemical-based deodorants.

Make-up – endocrine-disrupting chemicals are found in many cosmetics. They can interfere with hormones.

A perfume may contain up to 300 different fragrance chemicals called synthetic musks, which can cause extreme allergic reactions. Avoid alcohol perfumes with high alcohol content, which dry out the skin. Since many people spray it directly onto their necks, it can accelerate the formation of lines and wrinkles.

Beautiful, white teeth! They smile at us from everywhere: from posters, from magazines, from the television screen. We find them naturally attractive, for healthy teeth have always been regarded as an expression of vitality and beauty. In reality, preventive dental care and thorough oral hygiene have great significance that has long been overlooked. The texts of Ayurveda describe this holistic connection in detail. At the same time, they contain valuable recommendations, which should enable anyone to have healthy teeth throughout life, and fresh, pleasing breath. For example, the original texts state: 'Gargling with sesame oil is beneficial for the strength of jaws, depth of voice, flabbiness of face, excellent gustatory sensation and good taste for food. One [used to such gargles] never gets dryness of throat, nor do his lips ever get cracked. His teeth will never be carious and will be deep-rooted. His teeth can chew even the hardest foods.'

For this, take a tablespoonful of sesame oil, rinse the mouth with it briefly and then leave the oil in the mouth for three to four minutes to allow it to soak in between the teeth. Don't swallow the oil, which now contains toxins and harmful bacteria from the mouth, but spit it out. Rinsing the mouth purifies the whole mouth area, and if done regularly is said to be effective at preventing tooth decay and gum disease.

Ayurveda also recommends chewing aniseed and fennel seeds after meals. They not only have a cleansing and disinfectant action, they also taste good and stimulate digestion. A little time each day spent on your health may prevent a long time spent with illness.

Bad breath, or halitosis, may not be a serious medical condition but it can affect your personal comfort level. In most cases, it originates in the mouth and can be prevented right there. This potentially embarrassing problem is mainly caused by sulphur-producing bacteria that live within the surface of the tongue and throat. When these bacteria break down protein, they release a sulphurous odour resulting in bad breath. Other causes include dry mouth, gum problems, poor oral hygiene, post-nasal drip, certain medications, respiratory infections and particular foods. The following tips will help you take control over your exhalation.

Good oral hygiene is the most important factor in keeping your mouth and breath fresh. When you wake up in the morning you probably notice a white coating on your tongue that is the result of ama, the toxic waste-product of digestion. The best tool for removing the coating is a silver tongue scraper. Tongue cleaning is part of the ancient Ayurvedic tradition and widely practised in Eastern cultures. By removing the soft plaque from the tongue, especially the back of the tongue, you eliminate most of the bacteria that create the volatile sulphur compounds.

Brushing your teeth just after waking up, before going to bed, and at least once during the day after you eat will also help. Don't neglect to floss thoroughly once a day to clean the area between the teeth. Visit your dentist regularly to check for cavities, and have your teeth cleaned periodically by a dental professional.

To freshen your breath during the day, chew on mint leaves, cloves or fennel seeds. What you eat also affects the air you exhale. Certain foods, that already contain sulphur, contribute to the unpleasant odour. Once the food is absorbed into the bloodstream, it is transferred to the lungs where it is expelled. The odour will continue until the body eliminates food. The major culprits are onion and garlic. Try to avoid as many of these as you can, and clean your mouth after eating or drinking milk products. Animal protein and foods processed with sulphur additives, such as beer, wine and soft drinks, can also release odour. Smoking has been known to contribute to bad breath, discolouration of the teeth, and other mouth problems.

Dryness in the mouth means you don't have sufficient saliva flow that would help to remove bacteria and debris from the mouth. Breathing through the mouth, drinking alcohol and certain medications can be behind the problem. Try to eliminate the causes and drink plenty of water and herbal teas.

Other reasons for unpleasant breath can result from a variety of respiratory problems, such as upper respiratory allergies, infections of the respiratory tract (nose, throat, windpipe, lungs), chronic bronchitis, and chronic sinusitis. Constipation can influence your breath so you need to make sure your elimination is regular. Just as for cleaning the tongue, morning is the best time for elimination as well. For daily elimination drink plenty of water, eat lots of fresh vegetables and fruits, and add prunes and figs to your diet.

Oral cleanse – gargle with one tablespoon of warm sesame oil for five minutes, and do not swallow! Spit out the oil, and rinse your mouth with warm water. Then brush your teeth and gums thoroughly. Clean your tongue with a tongue scraper or firm toothbrush. Studies have shown people with gum disease often suffer atherosclerosis – blood-vessel narrowing that can cause heart attacks or a stroke. Maintaining oral hygiene requires flossing as well as brushing and gargling. In addition to brushing the teeth, Ayurveda puts great emphasis on gently scraping the top surface of the tongue in the morning to remove any deposits that may collect there overnight.

The number of household cleaning products and disinfectants containing antibacterial agents such as Triclosan is increasing. These agents have the potential to encourage bacterial resistance and general sickness and cause cancer.

Dry-cleaning uses a chemical called perc, which is believed to be carcinogenic (cancer causing).

Artificial lighting, concrete walls, central heating and computers all affect our energy levels. Slumping over a desk or lolling in a chair not only constricts your breathing, but also puts a drain on your energy resources.

Change your posture, sit or stand up straight, pull your shoulders back and allow your arms to hang loosely by your sides. Pull your stomach muscles in to support your spine, and try not to cross your legs.

Allow time for walks through your local park, spend time in your garden, and surround yourself with plants or window boxes. Get back to nature.

Shun smoking and other stimulants, as they will reintroduce toxins back into the body. Smoking not only causes lung cancer and many other cancers, but also contributes, very significantly, to a series of chronic diseases and conditions, including high blood pressure, high cholesterol levels, heart disease, emphysema, stomach ulcers, depression, anger-management problems and more. According to research carried out in Spain, mothers who smoke are 60% more likely than non-smoking mothers to give birth to a child with a defect.

Ayurveda recognises that breathing is one of the processes through which prana enters our system. As smoke-borne tars coat the alveoli (lung's air cells), the body's capacity to absorb oxygen diminishes. At the same time, the smoker's ability to assimilate prana dwindles.

If you woke up breathing this morning, congratulations, you have another chance. If you woke up this morning with more health than illness, you are more blessed than the million who won't survive the week (according to World Health Organisation figures). If you have food in your refrigerator, clothes on your back, a roof over your head and a place to sleep, you are richer than 75% of this world. If you have money in the bank, in your wallet, and spare change in a dish someplace, you are among the top 8% of the world's wealthy. If you hold up your head with a smile on your face and are truly thankful, you are blessed because the majority can, but most do not. If you can hold someone's hand, hug them or even touch them on the shoulder, you are blessed because you can offer a healing touch. If you can read this, you are more blessed than over two billion people in the world who cannot read anything at all. You are blessed in ways you may never even know.

Sleep

We have internal rhythms called circadian rhythms. These are set inside us all. We have a sleeping/waking rhythm that mirrors the day and night very closely. To be in optimum health we need to listen to that internal body clock. If we do not follow it, we can end up with fatigue or tiredness, which does not seem to go away. It has been found in experiments that most mistakes or accidents are made between midnight and 8.00am. This is when our bodies naturally want to be asleep. Seven to eight hours is usually said to be the amount of time needed for sleep.

Some very interesting things happen when we are asleep. This is the time when we are built up again and the events of life slip into perspective. We talk of needing to 'sleep on it', so we understand what this means. While we are asleep certain hormones are released into our bodies. The first is the growth hormone. This is produced in the hours before midnight, in the early part of our natural sleep cycle. It improves the size of the brain and body growth in the developing child. In adults, it aids the quality and efficiency of the brain and repairs damage to body tissue.

REMEMBER
Mothers who smoke are 60% more likely than non-smoking mothers to give birth to a child with a defect.

REMEMBER
When we breathe prana enters our system.

After this hormone has peaked, another is produced, called cortisol. This one peaks early in the morning. It goes to work on the membranes of the body and can also be an anti-stress hormone. A further hormone called melatonin is produced during the night and this is a natural tranquilliser. The old adage, 'early to bed and early to rise, makes a man or woman healthy, wealthy and wise,' would appear to have a considerable degree of truth in it. Shakespeare wrote of sleep 'knitting up the ravelled sleeve of care'. It is quite true that the frayed edges of our bodies are being knitted up again during this time.

Our brains have electrical waves that can be measured, and different ones occur at different times during the night. The deepest sleep occurs when we are having delta waves. These are long, slow, deep brain waves. In this sleep the cortex of our brain, where daytime conscious thought takes place, is recharged like a battery. During these times in the night our breathing is slow and deep, the heart rate slows down and our blood pressure drops. We are preparing chemically for another day of life.

There are other levels of sleep too. First, drowsiness, then another, a stage lower, where we are almost barely conscious of what is happening and then two average levels of sleep. But there is one other very interesting level of sleep. During this time we have rapid eye movements. It is sometimes called REM sleep. Brain waves speed up, the muscles become lax and soft, or make little jumpy movements, and blood pressure can rise. This is when we dream.

In this sleep the eyes are moving around all the time and it has been discovered that sometimes they do not even rotate together, but work independently of each other! So when we are dreaming we are not actually focussing on what we 'see'. This kind of sleep is important for us. Babies have 40–50% REM sleep; adults have a lot less.

Rest

Rest allows the body to heal and settle after treatment. Healing is a process that takes time. Your age, condition, lifestyle and willingness to follow Ayurvedic recommendations will affect the pace of your improvement.

Listen to your body. It will tell you when it needs an energy boost. If you're feeling sleepy, but it's still two hours before your usual bedtime, go with the message your body is telling you, rather than obeying the clock.

Take time to relax and combat the negative effects of stress. Engage in a gentle form of exercise for the mind and body, e.g. relaxation with breathing techniques, yoga, self-massage, nam-simran. Relaxation is very important in order to activate the inner healing forces of the body.

ACTIVITY

Research some relaxation exercises that could be given to the client to practise at home.

If you haven't exercised for a while, don't exercise too strenuously to begin with; overtired muscles create waste products and a strain on the lymphatic system. Whatever exercise you decide to do, begin slowly and then build up gradually. Don't push yourself too hard. Don't choose something you don't like – remember, exercise should be enjoyable.

Commit to better health. Use this opportunity to establish some new health habits. Each visit builds on the ones before. Frequency of future treatments and other related treatments ought to be encouraged for the maximum benefit.

Keep a positive outlook. Therapists are optimistic and clients should be too! Clients with a positive attitude heal faster. Find out what the client wants from the treatment. Present options for change, discuss barriers to change, help the client create a plan for change, confirm readiness and then help to change. Monitor progress and re-evaluate where necessary.

Do not waste energy with damagingly strong emotions. We have only one bank account of nervous energy. If you feel angry or frustrated or disappointed, is it worth becoming agitated? To do this is actually exhausting. It is better to turn away and think that there will always be another day. Strong emotions rarely change anything, and do not actually get back at the other person as we intend. They just tire us out. Remind clients to try and be calm, relax in a cool environment, and try to avoid confrontations, crowds, noise and heavy traffic.

REMEMBER
Encourage your client to keep a positive outlook.

Prime sources of toxins

- Aerosol body sprays
- Alcoholic beverages
- Caffeine
- Carbonated water
- Cigarettes and drugs
- Meat and fish

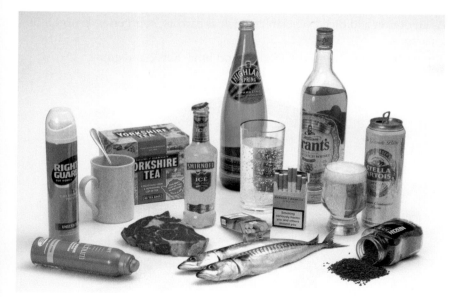

Fig. 12.05 *Toxins*

Here is a principle to remember:

- Morning – badhshah   Breakfast like a king,
- Noon – shasziada   Lunch like a prince,
- Afternoon – fakir   Tea like a pauper.

We need to be aware of the steps we can take that will improve our health, such as eating a healthy diet, stopping smoking and drinking and being more physically active.

Kitchari recipe

A light diet of kitchari would be useful to accompany the treatment, which can be taken again on the day after the treatment.

- Quarter of a cup of split yellow mung beans
- Quarter of a cup of white basmati rice
- 2 cups of water
- Quarter of an inch slice of fresh ginger
- Half a teaspoon of cumin powder
- Quarter of a cup of freshly chopped coriander leaves
- Half a teaspoon of turmeric powder
- One tablespoon of ghee (clarified butter)

Method

The mung beans do not need soaking in water.

Combine the rice with the mung beans and wash twice.

Bring the water to the boil in a saucepan.

Add the mung beans, basmati rice, fresh ginger and salt.

Cover and simmer on low heat for 30 minutes until tender, with a porridge-like consistency.

Melt the ghee in a saucepan.

Add the spices (cumin, salt and turmeric), stir until slightly browned.

Then mix into rice and beans.

Cook for about 20 minutes.

As an option add diced vegetables, such as carrots, courgettes, broccoli or asparagus.

Top with freshly chopped coriander and lime. Serve and enjoy.

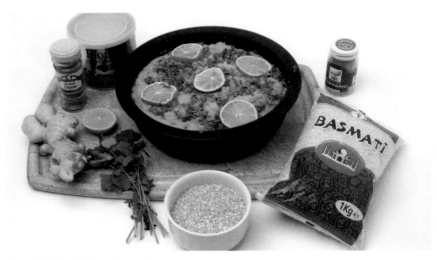

Fig. 12.06 *Kitchari ingredients*

1. State four food groups which are important to health.
2. Why should clients be encouraged to drink water?
3. Describe the three types of food found in Vedic scriptures: satvic, rajasic and tasmasic.
4. Describe the advice given to clients after treatment.

Key Terms

You need to know what these words mean. Go back through the chapter or check in the glossary to find out.

- Satvic
- Rajasic
- Tamasic
- Karma
- Rishis
- Triclosan
- Circadian rhythms
- Cortisol
- Kitchari

Business Matters

After working through this chapter you will be able to:

- Understand important health and safety aspects
- Learn about legal responsibilities and insurance
- Understand the importance of drafting a business plan and where to get help
- Understand your responsibilities for maintaining accounts, filing tax returns and paying National Insurance contributions
- Know how to contact advisory services or help-lines that can assist you in managing the business side of your Indian Head Massage practice.

Health and safety (related to the United Kingdom)

Health and Safety at Work Act, 1974

The Health and Safety at Work Act ensures that employers maintain high standards of health and safety in the workplace.

If an employer has more than five employees, the workplace must have a health and safety policy, which all staff must be aware of.

Employers and employees have responsibilities under this act. Employers must ensure the following:

- The workplace does not pose a risk to the health and safety of employees and clients.
- All equipment must be safe and have regular checks.
- There must be a safe system of cash handling, such as when taking money to the bank.
- Staff should be aware of safety procedures in the workplace and have the necessary information, instruction and training.

Employees' responsibilities include:

- To follow the health and safety policy.
- Read the hazard warning labels on containers and follow the advice.
- Report any potential hazard such as glass breakage or spillage of chemicals to the relevant person in the workplace.

The Health and Safety (First Aid) Regulations, 1981

A place of work must have a first-aid box containing the following: plasters, bandages, wound dressings, safety pins, eyepads and cleaning wipes.

When first aid is carried out, information such as the patient's name, date, place, time, events and any injury and treatment/advice given must be recorded.

> **REMEMBER**
> The Health and Safety at Work Act ensures that there are high standards of health and safety in the workplace.

Table 13.01 *Fire extinguishers are colour-coded for different types of fire*

Colour	Contents of fire extinguisher	Type of fire it is used for
Red	Water	Wood, paper, clothing, etc.
Blue	Dry powder	Flammable liquids (safe for electrical fires)
Cream	Foam	Flammable liquids (unsafe for electrical fires)
Black	Carbon dioxide (CO_2)	Flammable liquids (safe for electrical fires)
Green	Vapourising liquids	Flammable liquids (safe for electrical fires)

Fire Precautions Act, 1971

This Act states that all staff must be trained in fire and emergency evacuation procedure and that the premises must have fire escapes.

- There must be adequate fire-fighting equipment in good working order.
- Clearly marked fire exit doors must not be obstructed.
- Smoke alarms must be used.
- All staff must be trained in fire drill procedures and this information should be displayed at the workplace.

Control of Substances Hazardous to Health (COSHH), 1994

COSHH covers substances that can cause ill health. Hazardous substances such as essential oils must be used and stored away safely. All containers that contain potentially harmful chemicals must be clearly labelled. (Manufacturers often give safety information regarding their product.)

GOOD PRACTICE

Always read manufacturers' instructions regarding the storage, usage and disposal of substances.

Electricity at Work Act, 1989

This Act is concerned with safety while using electricity. Any electrical equipment must be checked regularly to ensure it is safe. All checks should be listed in a record book and could be important evidence in case of any legal action.

Reporting of Injuries, Diseases and Dangerous Occurrences Regulations (RIDDOR), 1995

Minor accidents should be entered into a record book, stating what occurred and what action was taken. Ideally, all concerned should sign. If as a result of an accident at work anyone is off work for more than three days, or someone is seriously injured, has a type of occupational disease certified by the doctor, or even dies, then the employer should send a report to the local authority environmental health department as soon as possible.

Employers' Liability Act, 1969

Employers must take out insurance policies in case of claims by employees for injury, disease or illness related to the workplace. The certificate must be displayed at work to show that the employer has this insurance.

REMEMBER

Advice regarding by-laws can be sought by contacting your local Environmental Health Officer.

By-laws

By-laws are laws made by your local council and are primarily concerned with hygiene practice. Different (town and city) councils around the country will have different by-laws. You will probably find there is not a by-law relating to Indian Head Massage treatment in your area.

Industry codes of practice for hygiene in salons and clinics

The code of practice is concerned with hygiene in the salon/clinic and gives guidelines for the therapist. Local by-laws contain these guidelines to ensure good hygienic practice and to avoid cross-infection.

Performing rights

Some practitioners like to play relaxing music while giving a treatment. Any music played in a waiting or treatment room is termed a public performance. If you play music you may need to purchase a licence from Phonographic Performance Ltd (PPL) or from the Performing Rights Society (PRS). These organisations collect the licence fees and give money to the performer and record companies. If you do not buy a licence, legal action may be taken against you.

However, many composers of music are not members of the PPL or PRS so no fee will need to be paid. To find out if you will need a licence contact the supplier of the music.

Data Protection Act

Any information about an individual, such as a client, that is stored on a computer must be registered with the data protection register. This Act ensures that this information is used by the practitioner only and not given to anyone else without the client's permission.

This Act does not apply to records stored manually, such as record cards stored in boxes.

The above information conforms to UK standards only.

Legal responsibilities

Table 13.02 *Insurance*

Employer's liability	Required if you employ people, in case of accident or injury to them whilst carrying out their duties
Public liability	Required to cover accident or injury to the public/client at your premises, or if you happen to cause your client injury whilst visiting them
Product liability	Required if you sell goods as part of your business, for any ill consequences deriving from the use of these products, e.g. oils, massage aids
Premises insurance	For fire and other damages, etc.
Loss of profit insurance	In case you are ill and cannot work
Asset insurance	E.g. massage table and other equipment, car if applicable
Personal accident or injury	Very important for the self-employed sole practitioner

Business insurance considerations for the therapist

Although insurance is something many people distrust or simply don't understand, it is vital when running a clinic to consider your package of protection and support against any possible financial vicissitudes in life. Insurance has offered valuable protection and support to many people for a very long period of time, and should be carefully considered, so that the same thoughtfulness and quality choices are made as in other areas of your practice.

GOOD PRACTICE

Ensure you have the relevant insurance when setting up in business.

Although this part may be a useful guide, there is no substitute for a skilled advisor, preferably specialising in insurance for health professionals, who can customise your package to suit your individual circumstances. Since 15 January 2005, all intermediaries are regulated by the Financial Services Authority by law, and are required to follow the strictest procedures, standards and practices.

Insurance is not only for the protection of you, the therapist, but also for your patients and the general public. Insurance is an essential factor in any business and is particularly relevant to practitioners in their contact with patients. Indeed, it is an integral aspect of professionalism and is particularly important in the current climate of greater recognition. More and more people are turning towards other approaches of health and healing, leading to greater exposure, and consequently a greater possibility of situations occurring or allegations of negligence against practitioners taking place.

With the advent of 'no win, no fee' solicitors, it is easier than ever to pursue a legal case. There are also disciplinary and complaint avenues for the public, which, since Statutory Regulation, are beginning to be used more and more. Furthermore, there is the ongoing harmonisation in the practice of Natural Medicine within the single European market.

There is a move towards greater quality control in areas of training standards, codes of conduct, ethics and insurance. In the past, insurance was seen as a necessary evil, or even not considered important, especially by a number of practitioners who relied on the fact that their type of therapy was safe, or that they had never had a claim in their career, or simply because they did not philosophically believe in it! Clearly this degree of naivety is no longer tenable or acceptable to the wider institutional world.

We will now explore some of the principal types of insurance that are relevant to you in setting up your treatment space, and protecting it against unforeseen mishaps which may arise.

Household insurance – working from home considerations

The standard householder policy will cover the building of your home or the contents for specific perils such as fire, lightning, storm damage, flooding, explosion, earthquake, aircraft, riot and civil commotion, malicious damage, theft and subsidence. Most policies offer an extension for accidental damage, to cover such things as staining, breaking, tearing and scratching insured items.

A word of warning for the therapist: the standard householder policy is intended for a home that is occupied residentially. Many insurance policies will not provide cover where there is business use, especially if members of the public are routinely coming in. Some insurers take the view that if the house is used for business purposes, the risk may well be increased. It is vital that insurers are advised of business use so that they cannot repudiate a claim because they were not informed. This is technically called a material non-disclosure.

It is very important that you advise your insurer and preferably obtain a satisfactory response in writing. There are now a number of policies which combine home and business coverage, but check these out before buying, as they can be a little inflexible and can be more expensive than a specialist practice-room policy combined with ordinary household insurance.

Practice-room combined packages

With household insurance for your furniture, equipment and stock, the first £50, £100 or even £250 typically may not be covered. This is known as the policy excess. There may be items of equipment that may be expensive and delicate in your clinic. These might be accidentally damaged, e.g. knocked over or broken. You need to ask your insurer for wider accidental damage cover if you possess any such equipment.

These policies also provide various other covers. There is public liability cover if, for example, a visiting client is injured while on the premises and where there is alleged negligence, giving rise to a legal liability on the part of the therapist. Also, employer's liability, which would cover any allegations of negligence causing injury to an employee, is available.

This insurance should also cover you for the loss of money in notes, coins and cheques on or off the premises for specific amounts. Loss of profits or increased cost of working cover, following property or contents damage, where the practice room is rendered unusable, and other optional covers, such as all risks for items in transit, or temporarily removed, can be covered.

Employer's liability

If you employ other staff, it is a legal requirement that you adopt employer's liability insurance. An employer's liability policy will meet the cost of any damages or other legal costs incurred where you, as the employer, have been held to be liable in some way.

REMEMBER
Employer's liability insurance is required if you have staff.

Typically, an employee could claim that the premises were unsafe or the equipment in the clinic had caused injury. Your policy will only provide cover if you are legally liable but there will be a generous limit of indemnity of £10 million for any one incident. If a payment is made to an employee, the damages awarded will relate to the seriousness of the injury and financial loss of the employee. Most practice-room packages include this, as mentioned above.

Public liability

Public liability is simply an insurance to protect the therapist against a claim from a member of the general public. Such policies usually have a limit of £1–2 million for any one payment. It is also known colloquially as 'trip and slip' cover. If a client were to trip over your carpet or fall down the stairs, he or she might be seriously injured. If a member of the public got hurt, the therapist could be sued for an allegation of negligence. A public liability policy enables the therapist to sleep peacefully at night, knowing that he or she would be fully protected if such an unfortunate and unforeseen accident occurred.

You have a responsibility to make sure that your premises are safe and any potentially hazardous items are not left lying around. The same applies if you rent rooms at a clinic or health centre. Although the owner may say that they have public liability cover, this will protect them if they are deemed legally liable, but not you. For example, you might be accused of damaging the room in some way, or your patient may be injured as a result of something you have done, so please don't rely on someone else's policy to protect you, as a number of therapists sometimes do!

GOOD PRACTICE

Regularly carry out a risk assessment at the workplace to ensure the safety of all who enter it.

Public liability with treatment risk extension

In the early days of specialist natural medicine insurance, the majority of policies to protect practitioners from claims were somewhat restricted in scope. Of these, the general public liability insurance, with a treatment risk extension tagged on to it, was the most commonly available. Some types of schemes, however, only cover a limited range of therapies.

Therapists who practise two or more therapies may find that they have to pay extra for the additional disciplines practised. Public liability with a treatment risk extension is often only valid either whilst the practitioner is treating, prescribing or advising a patient and normally covers the practitioner for incidents occurring in the year insured.

A major disadvantage is that they cannot be upgraded in future years, to safeguard the therapist for any (as yet) undiscovered claims, which may surface in the future when court awards are rising. These can sometimes leap up due to changes in case law, changes in interest rates for settlement damages cash awards that are invested, plus the fact that inflation has gradually eroded the value of the indemnity limit (typically £500,000 or £1 million), which applied to the year when the treatment took place.

> **REMEMBER**
> The general public are much more aware of their rights and will sue a therapist if the treatment they have received has in any way caused them injury, pain or suffering, or if there is a pure financial loss, allegation of breach of confidentiality, etc.

Professional indemnity

In this day and age, the treatment risk extension is simply not adequate. The general public are much more aware of their rights and will sue a therapist if the treatment they have received has in any way caused them injury, pain or suffering, or if there is a pure financial loss, allegation of breach of confidentiality, etc. In an era of increasing competition amongst therapists, allegations of libel or slander may arise not only from patients or clients, but also from other practitioners or teachers.

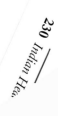

Under the statute of limitation, if someone wishes to sue you they have to initiate proceedings within a three-year period of the date of discovery for injury claims, or six years for damage or financial loss claims. In the case of a minor, these limits apply after the age of majority (18).

Therapists can now opt to cover their professional indemnity and malpractice insurance at a relatively inexpensive price. While covers used to be expensive, the growth of the natural medicine market has ensured a more competitive marketplace and specialist covers have been developed.

REMEMBER
Professional indemnity insurance is practitioner based rather than therapy based, and covers risks associated with behaviour as well as treatment.

Professional indemnity insurance is practitioner based rather than therapy based, and covers risks associated with behaviour as well as treatment. A good policy should insure the therapist for full professional indemnity risks, as well as public liability referred to above, and product cover, referred to later. The policy should cover more than one clinic where appropriate, and be flexible enough to include all of your therapies. The insurers normally require copies of certificates or qualifications, and the premium will be based on classification of risk and the number of therapies. Premiums for therapies involving manipulation will be more expensive than for counselling.

Unlike most policies you may be familiar with, which provide cover for the damage at the time it occurs, professional indemnity policies provide cover at the time when a potential claim is reported to or discovered by the therapist. Thus, a current policy would provide cover in respect of treatment carried out some years previously, but when the client has only now reported injury.

It is important when you effect a malpractice policy to agree with the insurers the number of years that you have been practising, for which they will now meet a claim. The technical term is the retroactive date. When you terminate the policy you will need to arrange 'run-off' cover to ensure that you are covered for any subsequent claims, until you are clear of the statute of limitation period. Many of the best policies currently available automatically include these clauses.

You should also appreciate that liability and indemnity policies normally only cover civil liability or negligence. Allegations of criminal negligence and allegations of sexual impropriety, for example, would not be covered unless you have a specialist legal cover for these types of situation. It is important to check whether a policy covers you for criminal allegations as well as negligence.

Malpractice

What can I do to lessen the likelihood of a complaint or successful action against me for malpractice? Consumers are becoming more aware of their legal rights and how to exercise them in the courts should the need arise. The situation is being aggravated by the new breed of legal firms who advertise 'no win, no fee' services, and encourage people that they might be able to collect thousands of pounds in compensation. These attempts, whether unfounded or not, are definitely on the increase, as are allegations of sexual impropriety and assault.

Here are some relevant points and a few basic precautions you can take to avoid situations occurring:

♦ Do not display your insurance certificate on the wall. For some people it may be an open invitation to claim, and you could be prejudicing your insurers.

- Many policy conditions state you should make client records and keep them for seven years. In fact you should keep them longer than that, particularly in respect of younger clients (children), where the statute of limitation states that a claim could be brought against you up to three years after reaching the age of majority (18).
- Your client's notes are a main source of defence – make sure that they are intelligible to others and always keep them in a safe place, preferably locked. Avoid assumptions or inferences and stick to observed facts. Any alterations if in your own hand should be crossed out and initialled/dated. Confidentiality and data-protection issues should always be considered.
- You must notify your insurance brokers, within 30 days of any circumstance that may give rise to a claim. Always declare previous incidents on any forms you have to complete when starting or renewing cover, even though you think the underwriter may already know about them. Do not enter into dialogue or correspondence about the complaint. Insurers may decline a claim if you do not comply with policy terms and conditions.
- Take care when advertising and in conversation, that no claims for cure are made. Even anecdotal conversations about your previous successes may be interpreted wrongly.
- A number of complaints seem to flow from misunderstandings or communications issues, and a failure to establish a good-quality therapeutic relationship.
- Refer to another healthcare practitioner when appropriate, particularly if a condition or situation is beyond the scope of what you have been trained to do, or where you may feel out of your depth.
- Extra care needs to be taken with children, particularly if they are experiencing headaches or high temperatures.
- If you are a multi-therapist and you decide to employ a different therapy from the one that your patient came for, involve the patient in that decision and ensure that your client is in agreement. Make sure that the client notes reflect this process and can be followed.
- For techniques involving contact in erogenous zones, make sure that you have explained this and obtained the client's permission, preferably written, and/or offer a chaperone. Record this in the notes.

> **REMEMBER**
> It is important to build a good rapport with your clients.

How do you recognise a medical malpractice claim? Many situations can be regarded as potential claims, before they are actually made against you, either directly in writing or via a solicitor. It is important that the warning signs are noticed and acted upon as soon as possible, to reduce the chances of a claim developing further, with the consequent stress and possible effect on your reputation. It is understood that you may not be negligent – the cover is there to help you clear your name if innocent, or deal with the expenses and costs if you are found to be negligent.

Danger signs include:

- Verbal complaint from a dissatisfied client, with a threat of taking things further.
- Letter of complaint alleging dissatisfaction, neglect, error or omission.
- A client not showing up for a subsequent treatment without explanation or further contact.
- A client or patient refusing to settle or delaying settlement of your account for an unreasonable period.

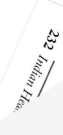

♦ A request for a refund of fees because the treatment has not worked or met with expectations, or is stated as having caused harm in some way.

Product liability insurance

If you make up, or simply supply any of your own or other people's products or remedies, you should ensure your policy provides product liability cover. This covers any legal liability following injury caused to anyone as a result of a defect in the product or remedy.

Most policies will not cover a defect in the formulation of the remedy if sold on a retail basis, where there is no client/therapist relationship. Under an EU directive, you are held liable even if you innocently supplied the defective product. Some policies only cover you whilst supplying your own patients. If you retail these goods to people who are not your clients, you may need to arrange a separate policy.

What should I do if a patient complains?

Try not to panic or get defensive, maintain goodwill, but above all do not admit liability or indicate that you are insured. Your position will be weakened and it will make it more difficult for the insurers to successfully defend you.

These are difficult times and you may feel vulnerable and angry. After many years of study and successful practice, you may feel that your professional life will be jeopardised by adverse publicity or possible financial consequences. It is helpful to talk things over with sympathetic peers and with your insurance broker. Try not to worry or let the situation affect your work.

These situations take on many twists and turns, and many attempts to claim do actually peter out if the therapist works the process through, provided he/she follows the guidance of the insurers and the underwriters' representatives, and complies with the terms and conditions of the policies.

If the incident involves any possible criminal proceedings you should phone your legal helpline, if your policy has one. Do not make any offers, but contact your intermediary (and the helpline if appropriate). Do not try to defend yourself or get involved in correspondence or communications on your own account. Tactfully explain that you will reply when you have had time to consider the complaint further.

Some clinics have an in-house complaints procedure. This is a sign of good practice, but the procedure must be allowed to go hand in hand with your insurer's agreement at every stage. They should give initial and ongoing advice and support. A claims handler or solicitor may investigate on your behalf. Pass on any correspondence received unanswered. Send in your client notes and your response to the allegations. Try not to make any judgements as to whether the circumstances are valid or not; leave that to the insurers or their representatives. If in doubt – notify!

Preparing for the future

It is important to develop a strategy with your financial planning, and to break down your priorities into short-, medium- and long-term goals. You

> **REMEMBER**
> Any incorrect advice causing injury or damage emerging from the advice is covered under the malpractice or treatment risk policy.

> **REMEMBER**
> You must notify your insurers once you become aware of any situation which may result in a claim being made against you.

should realise that there is nothing to be afraid of in dealing with these matters, but should prudently keep some money in hand for any short-term emergencies.

Try to avoid stocks and shares, unless you have expertise and a substantial amount of money to invest. Collective or pooled investments, such as unit trusts, are more preferable for medium-term (four to six years) investment, as the risks are spread. Although past history shows that equities outperform all other forms of investment, these are not guaranteed, and the nature of the beast is that it is cyclical and goes up and down in waves. It depends when you buy and when you sell as to how much your capital has grown. Try not to spend all you earn, but keep money in reserve, so that your business has a capital base, and you do not have to borrow more than you have to when required, as this is inevitably expensive over the longer term.

Here are some of the main types of financial services products that are available:

Pensions

Those who are unable to join a company pension scheme, or who are self-employed, need to consider a personal pension plan. The Inland Revenue allows generous contributions limits – from 17.5% to 40% of taxable earnings – according to the age of the investor. Full tax relief is given to the individual and, for those who are employed, contributions are paid net of basic-rate tax relief. Higher-rate relief is obtained through the individual's coding. The self-employed now pay contributions net, with higher-rate tax relief being obtained at the end of the tax year. The Inland Revenue also allows financial institutions to invest pension funds largely free of income and capital gains tax, which improves the investment return available.

Although the majority of a personal pension fund should be converted into a pension when retirement age is reached, tax-free cash for personal use is now easier to extract, following a simplification in pension legislation, which takes effect in 2006. In the event of death before retirement, the full value of the policy may be used for the benefit of the next of kin.

Since April 2001, there is now no need to have taxable income to take out a pension and receive tax relief on it. Policies can be taken out for children, and up to the age of 75, when they have to be cashed.

Stakeholder pensions have also been launched, offering charges below 1% per annum, and no penalties for stopping, starting or transferring. These are good value, but some providers offer more investment choice, and therefore the potential for higher returns, which a stakeholder product may not offer.

Health insurance

There are four aspects to this:

1. Long-term disability insurance

Often known as permanent health insurance, it provides a regular income in the event of long-term disability due to illness or injury. Premiums are paid to insurance companies who guarantee to pay income to an employed or self-employed person whose disability lasts beyond a specified deferred period. Up to 60% of income can be insured in this way.

Once the waiting period is completed (typically one to three months), and provided medical evidence proves that a person cannot work, the insurance company will pay the employed or self-employed person an income as provided under the policy until such time as the individual returns to work, dies or reaches the specified termination age (usually their retirement age) in the policy.

Should the disabled person return to work part-time or in a lesser, lower-paid capacity, arrangements can usually be made for the benefit to be proportionately reduced but still payable until such time as full recovery and total return to work is achieved. The income is free of tax, but a claim is subject to proof of income prior to the claim, and a maximum of 60% of taxable income is the norm these days.

Policies can be inflation-linked when not claiming, to take account of inflation, and inflation-linked when claiming, so that the disability income does not suffer in a long-term claim. Some policies give an investment element. Policies can also be taken out to provide for business expenses and the provision of a locum, in order to protect your practice whilst you are off work.

2. Personal accident and illness insurance
This covers both temporary total and temporary partial disablement, for up to two years' benefit (rather than to retirement age). In addition, loss of use of limbs, faculties, joints, etc. are covered for lump-sum compensation in the event of an accident. Premiums are generally cheaper, but cover is annually renewable rather than permanent, and insurers can revise their terms and exclude any serious claims made from future payments.

Some policies only pay out at the end of the disablement period, or at the insurer's discretion. Others are more generous in their claims handling and pay at the end of the month. The premiums are not age-related (permanent health premiums are). Insurers are also more flexible in their underwriting if you have had a previous health condition. Some health insurers will decline to insure you or require an extra premium; accident and sickness insurers may simply just exclude the pre-existing conditions.

3. Private medical insurance
As the National Health Service frequently fails to provide a speedy service for non-urgent conditions, some people feel a need for private medical insurance. This covers costs of hospitalisation, operations, medicines, fees and outpatient costs, etc. Insurance companies, in an effort to provide sensible and reasonably priced plans for the general public, offer policies with an excess, i.e. the policyholder agrees to pay the first £50 or £100 of any claim. This can significantly reduce the premiums which will be payable.

Furthermore, some modern plans provide private medical insurance only if the waiting period for National Health treatment exceeds six weeks. There are policies available which offer cover for complementary medicine upon referral by a GP or a specialist.

REMEMBER
Therapists should shop around for the best option if they wish to take private medical insurance.

4. Critical illness cover

If a member of a family is stricken with a life-threatening condition, not only is the ability of that person to earn their living in jeopardy, but their whole lifestyle may have to be drastically altered, which may prove expensive. Critical illness insurance can provide the necessary funds to enable that adjustment to be made more easily. There are a wide range of illnesses and types of permanent disablement situations that are covered such as cancer, heart conditions, MS, etc. These days many people can go on to live many years, or go into remission, so this cover can be especially relevant if you are single and have no dependants, and is more appropriate than the traditionally vaunted life cover.

Where do you go for advice?

The advice and guidance that you receive has to be paid for! Advisors are regulated by law and are strictly controlled. They have to study and pass examinations before they can practise, as well as having years of experience behind them. The process involves taking a financial case history, taking into account your needs, goals and attitude to risk, which is then condensed into a plan of action for you. Since the passing of the Financial Services Act, 1986, the terms 'independent financial advice' and 'independent financial adviser' have more meaning than ever before. Many sources of financial advice exist, e.g. banks, building societies, insurance companies, etc., who offer their own life assurance, pension and investment products to the general public. There are other advisers who, although not employed by a large institution, are nevertheless tied to one and sell their products only.

Although those who represent one company are regulated under the Act and frequently offer a highly professional service, they are unable to give an investor access to the whole marketplace. If they are unable to meet a client's requirements from their own portfolio of contracts, however, they are legally obliged to recommend that their client contacts an independent financial adviser.

Though the above information conforms to UK standards much of it is conventional to North America and Ireland.

Exclusive to United States of America
Types of insurance

Some types of insurance are required by law, while others may just offer additional protection.

- Professional liability insurance – covers the therapist for actions in their massage practice
- Business personal property insurance – protects your business equipment (i.e. desk, table, computer etc.)
- Liability insurance – covers cost of injuries that occur on your property to business-related visitors
- Homeowners insurance – if working out of your home check to see what coverage exists for business-related injuries to guests in your home
- Health insurance – medical coverage for the therapist
- Disability insurance – safeguards the therapist if they are unable to work due to injury or illness

> **REMEMBER**
> The advice and guidance that you receive has to be paid for! Advisors are regulated by law and are strictly controlled.

- Workers' compensation – is required by law if the therapist has employees in their business. They may also conform to standards set by OSHA (Occupational Safety and Health Administration).

Client confidentiality

Most states have laws concerning the privacy, confidentiality and handling of health information. Massage therapists need to comply with the requirements of their specific state as well as be aware of the new federal regulations concerning privacy.

Although most massage therapists (unless they are billing insurance companies) are not considered covered entities under the new Health Insurance Portability and Accountability Act (HIPAA) that has been in place since April 2003, they are still required to maintain the privacy of every client's healthcare and his/her records.

The purpose of HIPAA is to:

- Give consumers the right to have access to their health information and control the inappropriate use of that information
- Attempt to improve the trust that consumers have in the healthcare system
- Create national standards for privacy of healthcare information, especially those which pertain to electronic transmission of information.

Exclusive to Canada
Insurance

Insurance needs for businesses vary greatly. It is best to choose an insurance agent or broker familiar with your size of business and, in particular, an agent familiar with your type of operation. If you don't have an insurance agent, it could be a wise decision to ask other business owners in your area to recommend one.

The following list is included to remind you not to overlook the complex areas of business insurance. It is best, however, to discuss your specific requirements with your insurance agent. If you own a small business, you may need some or all of the following types of insurance.

Basic insurance:

- Fire insurance (extended coverage on buildings and contents)
- Liability insurance
- Burglary protection (theft coverage)
- Dishonesty insurance (covers thefts by employees)
- Business-interruption insurance, which compensates for the income lost if your business is unable to operate for a period of time due to disaster-related damage
- Liability insurance, in case someone suffers an injury or damage because of something your business did or didn't do
- Errors and omissions coverage, if you are in the position of offering advice to clients
- Possibly life, health, and disability insurance, for both yourself and your employees

◆ Workers' compensation, should an employee become injured as a result of a job-related accident or suffer an illness attributable to a workplace cause.

Business matters (relating to the United Kingdom)

Gaining a qualification in professional Indian Head Massage is the first necessary step to a successful practice. Working with clients is the definitive goal and to achieve this takes a lot of initiative and hard work.

Most modalities within complementary and alternative medicine are now part of everyday life and are accepted more and more by the public. Therefore, opportunities for giving Indian Head Massage are multiplying. At the same time, there is increased competition as more therapists are trained.

Identify your preferred place and style of practice

The first thing you need to do is to decide where you want to establish your practice. In an increasingly demanding market the options are:

1. Work independently in your own private clinic or home
2. Work with other beauty or complementary therapists in a spa/clinic environment
3. Work in a general practice surgery, hospital, hospice or nursing home
4. Work in a recreation facility, health club, holiday centre or gym
5. Work as a freelance therapist offering Indian Head Massage at clients' premises.

It is possible in some areas to combine more than one of these. You may decide that you prefer to give some, or even all of your treatments voluntarily. Some Indian Head Massage therapists are in a position to donate their skills, for example to a local hospice. Many Indian Head Massage therapists like working from home while others have a practice based on corporation/home visits to clients.

Apart from being employed by a spa/clinic, it may be worth considering self-employed opportunities. If you are employed, your employer is responsible for National Insurance contributions, and for working out your tax as part of Pay As You Earn (PAYE). Health and safety regulations are also the employer's responsibility. However, while your money is not put at risk and you are not directly responsible for profits or losses, you may have little or no say in the running of the business.

If you are self-employed, you are responsible for taxes, contributions, health and safety, as well as capital risks, but you can also enjoy creating your own enterprise. You may also need to decide if you want to work full-time or only part-time. This will determine to what extent you promote yourself.

Drafting a business plan

Before setting yourself up in business it is a good idea to create a business plan. Even if you don't need to show it to a bank manager, it will encourage you to think realistically about what you need and do not need for your practice.

> **REMEMBER**
> Any bank will be able to advise you on drawing up a business plan. They usually require this as part of an application for a loan.

The information asked for on a business plan includes such things as:

- Your training, qualifications and experience
- A customer profile or idea of your target market
- Proposed charges or a comparison with competitors' charges
- Setting-up and running costs
- Projections about profits and income from the business
- Cash-flow statements and forecasts – a cash-flow forecast is a way of working out how much cash a business is likely to generate in a future period. After you have been in business, it can be calculated on the basis of past receipts and payments made on a regular basis. The cash flow itself is found in the difference between outgoings and receipts over a given period.

Some government agencies may also be able to help with setting up a new business. They can be accessed through the internet or local telephone directory.

> **REMEMBER**
> Some government agencies may also be able to help with setting up a new business.

Planning

When you are planning the start of your practice, remember that in a business sense practising Indian Head Massage involves more than just giving the treatment. In order to give the treatment you need to have secured such things as the worksite, transportation to work, possibly the equipment, and overheads involved in running a clinic, even if yours is only a proportional contribution. In addition, keeping client records, ordering supplies, paying bills and promoting your business through talks and advertisements takes a certain amount of administration time which must be allowed for in your overall concept.

Good practice

From the beginning, set up a regular routine for your business administration. Do your paperwork, whether client records or your accounts, on a regular basis.

As people who just want to give a caring treatment it is easy to resent such considerations as not part of the treatment. We must remember that we do these things in order to enable us to give treatments, not as an end in themselves.

Starting up

Once in business, you must notify:

- Your local tax office
- Your local social security office
- Customs and Excise, if your annual turnover is above a certain amount
- Your local Job Centre, if you are registered with one.

Maintaining accounts

If you are self-employed you need to keep full and accurate records of all your business transactions. These include:

- All income received
- All business expenses incurred
- Drawing for yourself

- Any loans put into the business
- Capital expenditure items.

This information is filed as an annual return with the Inland Revenue/Inland Revenue Service (IRS) every financial year. These may be examined at any time so must be carefully and accurately kept. Bear in mind that accounts may also be required for reasons unconnected with tax, for example by your bank, when considering an application for a business loan.

Income tax

Each year in April you will receive a tax return to fill in giving information on the year's earnings, any capital gains and your net profit (the amount left over after expenses and eligible deductions for the year).

Your allowance is calculated by the Inland Revenue on the basis of the information you supply them about your individual circumstances. The Inland Revenue will issue you with a Notice of Coding or tax code which gives the amount of money you can earn tax free and detailing what benefits have been deducted.

It is a good idea to set money aside regularly to cover your yearly tax bill. Information about tax assessments and filing returns can be obtained from your local Inland Revenue office, and many local accountants offer free advice on the basics.

National Insurance

Most people who work are liable to pay National Insurance contributions, unless they qualify for an exemption. Self-employed people are liable for two classes of contributions:

1. Class 2 (paid towards benefits, except unemployment)
2. Class 4 (paid on profit and gains). Unless you have either been excused payment because of low earnings or are a married woman or a widow with reduced liability, in which case you must pay Class 2

These can be paid either quarterly every 13 weeks, or by direct debit every month.

Employers are responsible for Class 1, earning-related contributions to the PAYE scheme. An employee can claim for sickness, invalidity, maternity, unemployment, and widow's benefit where appropriate, once enough contributions have accumulated.

VAT

Value Added Tax (VAT) is a government tax charged on most goods and services. Currently the rate is 17.5% for businesses with a taxable annual turnover of £54,000 or more. As giving Indian Head Massage is a service, it may be liable for VAT once the turnover from the business reaches the annual amount, in which case the business must be registered for VAT with the local office. A registration number will be issued and true and accurate records must be kept on all business transactions. Every three months it will be necessary to fill in a VAT return form, and where output tax exceeds input tax the difference will need to be paid to Customs and Excise.

> **REMEMBER**
> If your earnings exceed your tax allowances – the money you are allowed to earn each year before paying tax – you will be assessed and required to pay tax.

Advertising and promoting your practice

Planning is essential when deciding ways to advertise and promote your practice. Give some thought to what type of client you wish to attract, then you can make decisions about such things as the appropriate medium for advertisements, as well as the style, tone and presentation, so that you engage the audience's attention.

Consider the five or six most vital pieces of information that should appear in any form of advertising for Indian Head Massage. Promotion needs to be cost effective as well and there are usually local avenues of free advertising. There are many ways to promote yourself besides advertising. A few of these are included here.

- Offer to give one treatment free for every five treatments received.
- Offer treatments as birthday or festive presents, with an attractive card which announces the gift treatment and gives details about yourself and how to book.
- Write letters introducing yourself to local support groups.
- Offer to give talks and demonstrations.
- Participate in any local aesthetic/complementary medicine fairs, though you need to check these out first to see how suitable they are and how productive they might be. If there are no such events, think about organising one yourself with other local therapists.

Create a business card and stationery

Create a leaflet for distribution to the public. Research the best sites where you might leave your leaflets for free distribution.

Write to your local GP practice manager introducing yourself, explaining Indian Head Massage and offering to arrange a meeting to discuss how Indian Head Massage might be useful to their patients.

Restrict yourself to one or two conditions which are common and which usually respond well to Indian Head Massage, and offer to do a trial period giving treatment for these. Such treatment may save the practice money on their prescription bills.

When you open your practice room, and whenever you have something of new interest to the public, send a press release to the local papers to try and get them to cover the event. The press release should be very brief but contain essential information: your name, address and telephone number, time/date/address of the event, and a brief description of its nature, in such a way as to engage the interest of the editor. Try to find an interesting and new angle to your story.

Giving talks

Giving talks to local groups of interested people is a very good way of promoting your practice and increasing public awareness of Indian Head Massage. Begin to formulate ways of promoting your practice in the local community.

Understand the value of giving talks to the public on Indian Head Massage and the important elements involved in public speaking. There are many organisations and groups looking for speakers at their regular meetings. More doctors, nurses and midwives are becoming aware of the benefits of CAM therapies. They want to know more and might be interested to have you as a speaker to their local associations.

Plan ahead and organise

As in any other activity, planning ahead is important. Before you even begin to outline your idea, think about the kind of audience you have so you can direct the tone and level of the talk to them, to their interests and experience, as far as you can. Being able to tie the information in the talk to specific aspects of their lives gives it more value.

Think about any posters or other visual material you could bring that will help you illustrate your ideas. As well as simply talking about Indian Head Massage, consider what activities you might also include, such as a demonstration of the technique, how this would be organised, and whether you think it's appropriate to get members of the audience to practise a technique on each other.

When planning your talk, put yourself in the position of members of the audience and think up questions they might have about Indian Head Massage. Gear your talk to try to answer these questions.

For example, if there are other health professionals in the audience, they might be very concerned to know about levels of training and professionalism, as well as about Indian Head Massage itself. Remember that many may be potential clients so they will want to know about costs, confidentiality, what is actually involved and often simply whether treatment is painful. Be prepared to answer such questions.

Write down all the ideas that you want to cover, and then think through them again. Aim to have an introduction and conclusion to round off the talk, and decide in what order you want to discuss your ideas. Use headlines to highlight the main points and make some notes on the information in this order. It is perfectly acceptable to use notes when speaking. Before you give your first public talk, practise it on a friend or family member, or at least in front of a mirror. This will take out some of the anxiety about public speaking.

Giving talks to the public is daunting for many people, especially at first. It helps if you can start with small, familiar groups. The more talks you give the easier it becomes. But there is always likely to be the odd question that comes as a surprise. The best approach is to speak from your own experience, including your life experience in general. Give concrete, specific examples whenever possible, and above all, don't be worried about admitting when something is outside your experience. It is perfectly acceptable to admit this, though it is helpful if you can think of someone to refer the questioner to for the answer.

> **REMEMBER**
> When planning your talk, put yourself in the position of members of the audience and think up questions they might have about Indian Head Massage.

Progress Check

1. List five types of insurance policies.
2. Why is it important to maintain client confidentiality?
3. Why is it important to have a good business plan?
4. Name two ways in which you could get free advertising.

Key Terms

You need to know what these words mean. Go back through the chapter or check in the glossary to find out.

- Insurance
- Business plan
- Income tax
- Cash-flow forecast
- National Insurance
- VAT

Case Studies

Case study 1

Client: Josie
Gender: Female
Age: 49
Occupation: Post Office clerk

First treatment
Josie had a mastectomy almost a year ago, followed by chemotherapy. At her last visit she discussed this treatment with her hospital consultant and was told that Indian Head Massage would not be a problem.

Second treatment
Josie stated that she felt very relaxed, loved every minute of receiving the treatment, and slept very well afterwards.

Third treatment
Josie again stated that she felt great. Though she is menopausal, she feels her flushes have decreased in frequency.

Fourth treatment
Josie stated that after the hair loss post-chemotherapy, she feels that the Indian Head Massage has in fact speeded up her hair regrowth.

Case study 2

Client: Guramy
Gender: Female
Age: 40
Occupation: Airport catering manager

First treatment
During her consultation, Guramy said that she had pain in her upper back, which comes and goes. She also complained of constipation, disturbed sleep and often wakes up in the middle of the night. Guramy has had two miscarriages. She also has poor eating habits as she skips breakfast, has a light lunch and often a late dinner. After her first Indian Head Massage treatment, she said it felt great and was relaxing.

Second treatment
After the second treatment she said there was no feeling of pain in her upper back and that she was regularly drinking four glasses of water per day.

Third treatment
After the third treatment, Guramy said constipation was not a problem any more and that she was sleeping without interruptions.

Fourth treatment

After the fourth treatment Guramy said that she is feeling healthier, has improved her eating habits, does not skip her breakfast, is eating more fresh fruit and vegetables, and now drinks up to six glasses of water per day.

General comments

The Indian Head Massage treatments have helped her to change her lifestyle and mind style in smarter and healthier ways.

Case study 3

Client: Ranjit
Gender: Male
Age: 22
Occupation: Baggage handler

First treatment

Contraindications checked:

- Diabetes controlled
- Blood sugar level reading before the treatment: 14.1; after the treatment: 4.9
- Saw white and red colours towards the end of the treatment

Second treatment

Contraindications checked (how do you feel after your last treatment?):

- Fell asleep straight after the first treatment
- Blood sugar level reading before the treatment: 9; after the treatment: 6.6
- Saw white and orange colours, and reported feeling smothered in a divine feeling

Third treatment

Contraindications checked (how do you feel after your last treatment?):

- Totally relaxed and had forgotten sleeping was this good
- Blood sugar level reading before the treatment: 7.9; after the treatment: 5.4
- Receiving spiritual energy with the treatment

Fourth treatment

Contraindications checked (how do you feel after your last treatment?):

- Feeling wonderful, want this to continue for the rest of my life
- Blood sugar level reading before the treatment: 6.9; after the treatment: 5.5
- As he was insulin dependent, he was surprised by the blood test results after the Indian Head Massage

General comments

Results like these have never been achieved before by all the medication he has been given.

Case study 4

Client: Shirley
Gender: Female
Age: 31
Occupation: Housewife

First treatment
I found this very relaxing, it made me tingle all over, and I saw a white light. I felt tired and thirsty and a bit light-headed. In the morning, I ached slightly and felt groggy, but then I felt energised and realised I had had a very good night's sleep.

Second treatment
I felt that it all flowed together nicely and felt a lot more relaxed. I tingled all over most of the time the next day. I felt full of energy and mentally free and good about myself.

Third treatment
I felt light-headed and totally numb when finished. I saw the colour green during the treatment. But I felt really tired and relaxed after the treatment. I went home and laid on the bed where I saw, quite vividly, flashes of different stages of my life (good and bad). I was not sleeping or dreaming. The next day I felt great.

Fourth treatment
I felt extremely relaxed and saw white sparkling light turning purple around me after the treatment. As a sufferer of ME and CFS fibromyalgia, before my present treatments I had a bad sleeping pattern, ache in the muscles and generally felt quite ill and down.

General comments
Since having my Indian Head Massage, I can honestly say my life is changing. I have had no migraines and it has helped with my sleeping pattern. When I'm not having treatment on a regular basis. I feel as I used to before. I feel a lot more positive and healthy altogether. I have come on in leaps and bounds.

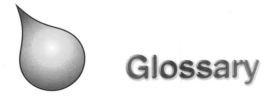

Glossary

Abhyanga: A daily therapeutic whole body oil massage to increase circulation, decrease dryness and reduce Vata aggravation.

Adipati: (1) A marma point also known as 'the lord of all' (marma points) situated on top of the cranium. Working on adipati controls sahasrar chakra, prana, srotas, vata, pita and kapa.

Adipose tissue: Fatty tissue, found between muscle fibres and under the skin, which gives the body a smooth, continuous outline. Also found around the kidneys and at the back of the eyes.

Adrenal gland: Situated one on top of each kidney, this gland secretes many hormones for different important functions, e.g. regulation of salts in the body; metabolism of carbohydrates, fats and proteins; sexual development, maturity and ovulation; and production of stress hormones to prepare the body for 'fight or flight' mechanism.

Agni: The fire element. The digestive fire, located in the gastrointestinal tract.

Agya chakra: Energy vortex at the third eye.

Akash: The element and universal organising principle of space.

Allopathy: Also known as the modern system of medicine, which treats a disease with pharmaceutical drugs.

Ama: The toxic residue of undigested food that is the source of illness in the body.

Aman: (2) A marma point situated between the thumb and index finger. Working on the aman controls headaches, certain srotas and avalambaka kapa.

Ambience: The perceived impression of a treatment room in relation to light, temperature, noise, appearance and atmosphere.

Amrit: Nectar.

Anagen: The first, growing, active phase of the hair growth cycle.

Anand: Bliss.

Anandamaya kosha: The spiritual body within the aura.

Annamaya kosha: The densest (physical) body within the aura.

Apana Prana: One of the five pranas. It is the prana that controls all evacuation, called the downward breath, and resides in the lower abdomen.

Apanga: (2) Marma points situated on both lateral sides of the orbital fossa. Working on apanga controls the sense organ of sight.

Aphrodisiac: Any substance that promotes the health of the reproductive organs.

Appendicular skeleton: This supports the appendages or limbs and attaches them to the rest of the body. It consists of the shoulder girdle, the upper limbs, the pelvic girdle and the lower limbs.

Arteries: Thick-walled, hollow tubes which carry oxygenated blood from the heart and veins and carry deoxygenated blood from the heart, except in the pulmonary system.

Asa: (1) Marma point situated at the third eye. Working on asa benefits the agya chakra and prana.

Asanas: Yoga postures designed to refine physiological functioning.

Asatya-Indi-Sanyog: The improper uses of the senses.

Ashram: Place devoted to spiritual development.

Astanga Hrdayam: One of the three ancient Ayurvedic texts of medicine.

Atma: Consciousness or God in an individualised sense.

Avtar: One of the manifestations of Vishnu, the force of preservation or organization in the universe.

Axial skeleton: This supports the head, neck and trunk (also known as the torso). It consists of the skull, the vertebral column, the ribs and the sternum.

Ayurveda: The science of life, the oldest health-care science known to man.

Basti: Therapeutic purification and rejuvenation of the colon. One of the five main procedures of panchakama.

Beeswax: Made by industrious honeybees from the nectar of flowers and prized since ancient times, beeswax candles burn longer and more cleanly than paraffin candles.

Bile: Bitter alkaline fluid, which aids digestion and is secreted by the liver and stored in the gall bladder.

Bio: Biological.

Brahma: Absolute consciousness; the aspect of consciousness in the divine trinity that is the creator or generator of each cosmos; the founder of Ayurveda in the form of god Dhanvantri.

Brahman: A term used to describe that which is not possible to describe; it is often just called being conscious, bliss, or sat, chit, anand; the self.

Bramand: Cosmic creation.

Brahma-acharya: Abidance in Brahma or the unmanifest reality.

Brimhana: Strengthening or fortifying therapies in Ayurveda.

Business plan: A document which details the business you hope to start and the expectations you have for its success for at least the first year.

CAM: Complementary and alternative medicine.

Capillaries: The smallest blood vessels which distribute essential oxygen and nutrients to most parts of the body.

Cardiac muscle: Only exists in the heart, and powers its pump action.

Cash-flow forecast: Prediction of net savings or profits that will accrue from earnings in a given time.

Catogen: The second, changing phase of the hair growth cycle.

Cells: The smallest unit of matter that can live independently and reproduce itself.

Central nervous system: One of two parts of the nervous system, consisting of the brain and the spinal cord, both covered by meninges.

Chakra: Energy vortex.

Charaka Samhita: The oldest surviving text of Ayurveda; one of the three ancient Ayurveda texts of medicine.

Chi: Chinese word for Prana.

Chit: Consciousness.

Client care: Taking care of a client by making them comfortable before and during their treatment.

Consciousness: As used in this book, the Source of all manifestation.

Consultation: An appointment between the therapist and a potential client before any treatment is given. This allows the therapist to give information about the treatment, for the client to voice any queries and questions they may have, and finally to ascertain if he or she is suitable for treatment.

Contra-action: A reaction to treatment.

Cortisol: A corticosteroid hormone produced by the adrenal cortex that is involved in the response to stress. It increases blood pressure and blood sugar levels, may cause infertility in women, and suppresses the immune system. Synthetic cortisol, also known as hydrocortisone, is used as a drug mainly to fight allergies and inflammation.

Cross-infection: The transmission of disease from one person to another.

Crystalline: Clear as crystal.

Dhatus: Tissue; one of the seven retainable substances or structures of the body.

Dhatu	Tissue
Rasa	plasma or nutrient fluid
Rakta	blood
Mamsa	muscle
Meda	bodily (adipose tissue)
Ashti	bone
Majja	bone marrow
Shukra	reproduction

Dermis: Also known as 'true skin', this layer sits under the epidermis and is connected to the blood and lymph supply, as well as nerves. Contains connective tissue as well as white collagen fibres and yellow elastic tissue known as elastin.

Dharm: Life's purpose (dharma).

Digestion: The breakdown and transformation of solid and liquid food into microscopic substances.

Dosha: Sanskrit for humour; literally that which will imbalance or 'fault'; a unique concept to describe the functions of the body; the forces, which balance the five elements together in the body. There are three humours: Vata (wind), Pita (fire) and Kapa (water).

Effleurage: Soothing, smooth stroking movements, performed with the whole palmar surface of the hand.

Employment standards: Work ethics and regime.

Endocrine: Secreting directly in to the blood.

Energetic impressions: In Sanskrit there are two kinds:

Vasanas: these are latent, unconscious, or stored impressions and current mental impressions.

Samskaras: these impressions are stored in the subtle body. Yoga says that these impressions are what cause us to incarnate in another life. Unless they are allowed to surface to consciousness, these impressions along with Prana create what we call mind.

Epidermis: The outermost layer of skin.

Esoteric: Doctrine.

Ethics: A set of moral values held by an individual or a group.

Friction: Deep pressure movements which can be performed in a small circular movement or transversely, across the muscle, pressing down on the underlying structures.

Gandharav Vidya: Ancient Indian form of music therapy, designed to restore physiological harmony and eliminate pathogenic imbalances.

Ghee: Purified butter.

Guru: Gu = ignorance Ru = enlightenment.

Healing space: Where peace, quietness, stillness, serenity and a smile would make you welcome.

Homeostasis: To work well the body systems need the right conditions for tissues and cells to function properly. Homeostasis is the means by which these internal body conditions are kept constant. Among the most important things the body needs to regulate are temperature; water and salt levels; and the amount of glucose in the blood.

Hygiene: It is the maintenance of healthy practices. Good hygiene is an aid to health, beauty, comfort, and social interactions. It directly aids in disease prevention and/or disease isolation.

Income tax: A tax paid on income.

Insurance: Provides protection and support against any possible unexpected financial changes in a practitioner's professional life.

Interface: Common boundary between two regions.

Involuntary muscles: These are muscles we do not consciously control.

Jal: The element and universal organising principle of liquid.

Kapa: One of the three doshas; controls water and earth elements.

Karma: Actions. The cosmic law that for every action there is a reaction.

Karna Purana: The application of oil in the ears.

Ki: Japanese word for Prana.

Kitchari: A mixture of basmati rice and split yellow mung dal, used to cleanse and balance the doshas during panchakarma therapy.

Krikatika: (2) Marma points situated on both sides of the joint of the head and the neck. Working on krikatika controls posture and alleviates pain in the back of the head and neck tension.

Krkara: A secondary prana that controls digestion.

Kundalini: The primordial Prana that rests dormant in the body unless activated by special practices.

Kurma: A secondary prana that controls the opening and closing of the eyes.

lanugo: Hairs that are found on the unborn child and are shed soon after or before birth. Lanugo hair is very soft and lacks pigmentation.

Latent impression: See Energetic impressions.

Life force: Another name of Prana.

Linga: Symptoms, shape, identification.

Lymph: A fluid, similar to blood plasma, that transports excess waste away from tissues.

Lymphatic node: Lymph vessels open up into lymph nodes which filter the lymph and remove and destroy harmful micro-organisms, tumour cells, and damaged or dead tissue cells.

Lymphatic vessel: These are vessels which transport lymph around the lymphatic system.

Mahabhutas: The universal organising principles which structure and govern all physical phenomena.

Mala: The natural metabolic by-products which are always eliminated from the body.

Manipur chakra: The solar plexus; the seat of fire within the body.

Manomaya kosha: The mental body within the aura.

Mantra: The science of sound. By using the correct sound each Prana can be harmonised, as well as the mind.

Marma: A nadi junction (sensitive point of the body that stimulates the pranic flow).

Massage: To rub and manipulate muscles and joints of the body to stimulate their actions.

Maya: The illusion that everything exists as separate from consciousness.

Meditation: To bring the mind and body into a state of stillness.

Mind: Thoughts moving through consciousness, giving the illusion of continuity; the combination of prana and vasanas.

Mooladhar chakra: Energy vortex between the anus and the genitalia.

Moong: Split yellow dal - lentil soup.

Multi-dimensional human system: Composition of Annamaya, Pranamaya Manomaya, Vijnanamaya, and Anandamaya.

Naad Brahma: Naad means sound and brahma means the cosmos. The state of the Cosmic Soul is sound.

Nadis: The channels of Prana in the body, meridians.

Nam-simran: Mantra-meditation.

Nasa: Nose.

Nasya: The application of medicinal oil in the nostrils.

National Insurance: A tax paid from wages to finance state benefits.

Netra Basti: Dispensing medicated ghee over the eyes in a retainer.

Nila: (2) A marma point situated at the junction of collarbone and sternum. Working on nila controls thyroid and bhrajaka pita.

No-mind: Non-movement of thought; complete awareness. Not to be confused with the Absolute - the individual may still exist at this point, it may take many times of being emerged in no-mind before the individual dissolves into pure consciousness.

Ojas: The most refined product of dhatu metabolism which controls the body's immune function.

Ovaries: Situated either side of the uterus, they are responsible for female sexual characteristics by secreting female sexual hormones.

Palmplan: Five elements, relating to each finger and thumb of the practitioner, that affect the internal organs of the client.

Panchamahabhuta: The theory of the five elements.

Panchakarma: The five actions; five reducing therapies in Ayurveda.

Paradigm: Pattern.

Param Atma: The universal intelligence of nature.

Parathyroid gland: There are four of these glands situated on either side behind the thyroid gland. They secrete hormones to help maintain calcium levels in plasma as well as its reabsorbtion into the kidneys.

Peripheral nervous system: One of two parts of the nervous system, consisting of the cranial and spinal nerves and the autonomic nervous system, which supplies nerves to all the body's internal organs.

Pétrissage: Pressure manipulation which includes kneading, picking up, wringing, rolling and friction.

Pita: One of the three humours; controls fire and water elements.

Pituitary gland: Situated behind the nose, it consists of the anterior (front) and the posterior (back) lobes. The anterior lobe produces hormones that control the endocrine glands and other body systems. The posterior lobe produces two main hormones that have an effect on the kidneys and the reproductive organs in females. Also known as the 'master gland' because of its controlling effect on the other glands.

Platelets: Irregularly shaped, colourless bodies that are present in blood. Their sticky surface lets them, along with other substances, form clots to stop bleeding.

Portal: Gate.

Pradhamana Nasya: The application of medicated powders in the nostrils.

Prakriti: The dynamic energy of consciousness; natal constitution; nature.

Prana: The vital force; vayu. It arises from substratum of pure consciousness with intelligence (agni) and love (soma). Together they create the individualised consciousness. There are five primary Pranas in the human body: apana, samana, udana, vayu and vyana.

Five minor Pranas:
Naga: Administers hiccupping.
Kurma: Administers opening and closing eyes.
Krkara: Administers digestion.
Devadatta: Administers yawning.
Dhanamjaya: Holds the body together after clinical death.

Pranamaya kosha: The etheric body within the aura.

Prana Vayu: The sub-dosha of vata, which governs sensory function and the intake of prana, water and food.

Pranayama: An alternate nostril breathing exercise, which increases the intake of prana.

Prithvi: The element and universal organising principle of form and structure. Also commonly known as the earth element.

Professional appearance: To present a professional image to the general public. A therapist should ensure that personal presentation is in line with public expectations.

Pulse: The rate at which the heart pumps blood through the circulatory system.

Purusha: The unmanifest aspect of consciousness; the void.

Qi: Chinese word for Prana.

Rajas: One of three gunas; actions, movement, energy aggressions, aggravated mind, achievement and strong emotions.

Raktamokshana: Therapeutic withdrawal of blood. One of the five major purificatory procedures of panchakarma.

Ram: Avtar; one of the manifestations of Vishnu, the force of preservation in the universe; the hero of the epic poem Ramayana; pure consciousness embodied.

Rasayana: One of the branches of Ayurvedic science having to do with Rejuvenation.

Red blood cells: They are the most common type of blood cell and are the body's principal means of delivering oxygen from the lungs to body tissues via the blood. Red blood cells are also known as erythrocytes.

Rishi: Sage, oracle.

Sacrament: A formal religious ceremony conferring a specific grace on those who receive it.

Sahasrar chakra: Energy vortex above the crown.

Samana Prana: One of the five Pranas in the body. Called the equalising prana, it resides in the navel region.

Samsara: The concept that we are separate from God; suffering; illusion.

Samskaras: Innate energetic impressions; see energetic impressions.

Sanskrit: The language of the Vedas from which Ayurveda comes.

Sat: Truth.

Satva: One of the three gunas; purity, peace, calm, beauty, happiness, quiet obedient mind and stable emotions.

Scalp oil massage: Stimulates the flow of blood to the follicles, bringing the nutrients necessary for a healthy scalp and harmonising doshas.

Self: Another name for pure consciousness. Also called Brahman or the substratum of all duality – i.e. creation; our true nature, hence the term – 'self'.

Shakha: Branch.

Shakti: Female cosmic Prana.

Shalyakya Tantra: This branch of Ayurveda medicine is dedicated to diseases located above the neck.

Shankha: (2) Marma points situated in between the tragus of the ear and the lateral corner of the eye. Working on shankha controls sense organs of touch and vata in the large intestine.

Shiro-Abhyanga: Traditional Indian Head Massage.

Shiva: Absolute consciousness; the aspect of consciousness in the divine trinity that is responsible for bringing each cosmos/life to its end.

Shringataka Lower: (1) A marma point situated at the centre of the chin crease. Working on Shringataka Lower controls prana, bodhaka kapa and the sense organ of taste.

Shringataka Upper: (1) a marma point situated at the centre of the chin crease. Working on shringataka Lower controls prana, bodhaka kapa and sense organ of taste.

Sidhi: Extrasensory perception.

Simanta: (4) Marma points situated at the corner of the forehead and temple region. Working on simanta controls majavaha, rasavaha and raktavaha srotas.

Siramatrika: (8) Marma points situated along the base of the occipital ridge. Working on the siramatrika benefits facial and jaw muscles and aids the clearing of middle-ear congestion.

Soma: Nectar; the most subtle essence of ojas and kapa.

Srotas: Channels in the Ayurvedic system that carry substances like blood, air and thought.

Stapani: (1) a marma point situated in between the eyebrows at the position of the third eye. Working on the stapani marma point benefits the agya chakra and prana.

Substratum: Equal to the Absolute, pure consciousness, love, Brahman, Atma, Self or Source.

Sushruta Samhita: One of the three ancient Ayurvedic texts of medicine.

Svedana: One of the two main purvakarma (preparatory procedures of panchkarma).

Tamas: One of the three gunas: inertia, dullness, depression, emptiness, laziness, despair and self-destructive emotions.

Tantra: A path that totally accepts all aspects of physical world, believing that all things lead to the divine; worship of the divine mother. Often confused with a sexual practice.

Tapotement: Stimulating percussion movements, which include hacking, clapping or cupping, beating and pounding.

Tejas: The subtle form of pita; the power of discrimination in the mind.

Telogen: The third and final resting phase of the hair growth cycle.

Terminal: Hairs are deep-rooted, well-developed, and coarse. Pigmented hairs replace lanugo and vellus hair. Terminal hair is found on the scalp, under the arms, and in the pubic region as well as on some other parts of the body.

Testes: Situated within the scrotum behind the penis, they are responsible for male sexual characteristics by secreting male sex hormones.

Thyroid gland: Situated either side of the neck, it secretes hormones to stimulate tissue metabolism and maintain BMR (basic metabolic rate).

Treatment plan: It is common practise to work with a treatment plan in order to record findings associated with each treatment.

Triclosan: A potent wide spectrum antibacterial and antifungal agent. It is found in soaps, deodorants, toothpaste and is impregnated in an increasing number of consumer products.

Tri-Doshas: Tri = three, Doshas = dynamic forces that determine growth and decay in the body and mind.

Tri-Gunas: Tri = three, Guna=quality. The attribute of intelligence; satva, rajas and tamas; the three phases of activity in creation as well as the three qualities of the mind.

Trikutu: A famous Ayurvedic formula that stimulates digestion and agni; very good for kapa.

Triphala: A famous Ayurvedic formula for rejuvenating the body, promoting digestion, and harmonising all the digestive organs.

Triple heater: A nadi called triple heater in oriental medicine that governs adrenal glands. In Ayurveda the adrenal glands in turn govern Pita.

Udana prana: One of the five pranas in the body, called the upward moving breath.

Upanishad: Spiritual interpretations on the Vedas. Their language is Sanskrit.

Utkshepa: (2) Marma points situated behind the upper border of the helix of the ear. Working on Utkshepa controls Vata and the sense organ of smell.

Vagabhata: A major commentator on Ayurvedic science after Charka and Sushruta.

Vaid: An Ayurvedic physician.

Vasanas: Latent energetic impression; see energetic impressions.

Vasishta: One of the seven immortal seers in the three ancient Ayurveda texts of medicine.

VAT: Value added tax.

Vata: One of three humours; controls wind (air) and space elements.

Vayu: The God of Wind; another name for Vata; another name for Prana.

Vedas: Literally means knowledge, the oldest book in the world; there are four almanacs.

Vedic lifestyle: Conscious living.

Veins: These carry deoxygenated blood back to the heart, apart from the pulmonary vein.

Vellus: Soft fine hairs, sometimes called down, covering most parts of the body except the palms of hands, soles of feet, lips and genital areas. Vellus hairs replace lanugo hairs and are classed as primary hairs.

Vibrations: Fine trembling movements, made using the whole palmar surface of the hand or with the fingertips only.

Vidhuru: (2) Marma points situated just below the mastoid bone. Working on Vidhuru controls functions for the sense organ of hearing.

Vijnanamaya kosha: The astral body within the aura.

Vikriti: Deviation from the original proportion of the tri-dohsa (prakriti).

Vikruti: The imbalance in the dosha that obscures one's parkurti or natal constitutional balance.

Vishnu: Absolute consciousness; the aspect of consciousness in the divine trinity that protects, organizes and preserves the cosmos; god Ram and god Krishna are the two most famous incarnations of Vishnu.

Voluntary muscles: These are the muscles which we consciously control, e.g. our arms and legs.

Vyana prana: One of the five pranas in the body. Called the equalising breath, it unifies all the other pranas and the body; it is diffused throughout the body.

White blood cells: Also known as leukocytes, these are cells which form a component of the blood. They are produced in the bone marrow and help to defend the body against infectious diseases and foreign materials as part of the immune system.

Yantra: A sound or syllable transformed into a geometric form, usually inscribed in a metal plate or in stone.

Yoga: Union. That which leads one back to the original Source.

Resource Directory for Training in Indian Head Massage

Please visit www.indianheadmassage.org for authentic training in Shiro-Abhyanga

United Kingdom

Atma Institute
PO Box 1, Windsor SL4 4 UZ
Tel: 01753 831 841
ayurvedicbodywork@yahoo.com

Urban Chill
22 Bloomsbury St, London WC1B 3QJ
Tel: 020 7267 8009
mark@urban-chill.com

VEBA
34 Langridge Dr, Brighton BN41 2JB
Tel: 01273 421 077
valdargonne@yahoo.com

Bristol School of Holistic Therapies
14 Orchard Street, Bristol BS1 5EH
Tel: 0870 889 0350
enquiries@bristolschoolofholistictherapies.co.uk

SM Cosmetics
32 Malmesbury Rd, Cheltenham GL51 9PL
Tel: 01242 570 515
susannah@smcfirst.com
www.smcfirst.com

Central YMCA Club
112 Gt Russell St, London WC1B 3NQ
Tel: 0207 343 1844
p.jelly@centralymca.org.uk
www.centralymca.org.uk

Bristol School of Spiritual Knowledge
5 Humber Place, Hull HU1 1UD
Tel: 01482 620 337
angie@bssk.co.uk
www.bssk.co.uk

The workshop at BHS
43 Ducie Road, Barton Hill, Bristol BS5 0AX
linnyj@bartonhillsettlement.org.uk
www.bartonhillsettlement.org.uk

City and Guilds
Customer Relations
1 Giltspur Street, London EC1A 9DD
Tel: +44(0) 207 294 2800
www.city-and-guilds.co.uk

VTCT
3rd Floor, Eastleigh House
Upper Market Street, Eastleigh, Hampshire S050 9FD
www.vtct.org.uk
customerservice@vtct.org.uk

ITEC
2nd Floor, Chiswick Gate
598-608 Chiswick High Road, London W4 5RT
Tel: +44(0) 20 8994 4141
www.itecworld.co.uk
intro@itecworld.co.uk

The Holistic and Beauty Academy
102b Soundwell Road, Staple Hill, Bristol, BS16 4RE
Tel: 01454 851754
www.holistic-training.co.uk

Ireland

Atma Institute Ireland
ayurvedictraining@hotmail.com

Obus School
53 Beech Gr, Lucan, Co Dublin, Ireland
Tel: 01628 2121
info@aromatherapytraining.com
www.aromatherapytraining.com

United States of America

American Inst of IHM
PO Box 963, Williamstown, NJ, 08094
Tel: +1 609 221 6513
ihm.usa@verizon.net

Canada

Canadian Inst of IHM
Tel: 250 729 4917 (Alberta)
ayurvedicbodywork@gmail.com

Tel: 780 430 8643 (Ontario)
nadineleah@hotmail.com

References

Aurobindo, Sri (1993) *The Integral Yoga: Sri Aurobindo's Teaching & Method of Practice*, Lotus Press, Twin Lakes, Wisconsin.

Evans, F.J. (1974) *The placebo response in pain reduction*. In J.J. Bonica (Ed.), *Advances in Neurology*, 289–296, Raven, New York.

Melhuish, A. (1978) *Executive Health*, London Business Books, London.

Quick and Quick (1984) to be confirmed

Index

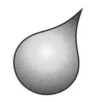

Page numbers in *italics* indicate figures or tables.

rest 221
rheumatoid arthritis 108, 135
ribosomes 47
ringworm 133, 135
Rishis 216, *216*
RSI (repetitive strain injuries) 100

SAD (seasonal affective disorder) 108
sage 145–6
Sahasrar chakra *36*, *37*, *39*, 197–9,
    197–9
Samana 22
Satva 17
    satvic diet 209, *210*
    satvic mind 25, 26, *27*
    satvic touch 156
scabies 133
scalp *90*, 91, 163
    care 215–17
    infections 135
    oil massage 149, 187–90, *187–90*
scar tissue 135
scleroderma 108
scoliosis 85, *85*
seasonal affective disorder (SAD) 108
sebaceous glands 62
sesame oil 150, 217
shakha marma points 195, *195*
Shalyakya Tantra 92
shampooing technique 189, *189*
shiro basti 44
Shiro-Abhyanga *see* Indian Head
    Massage
shirodhara 44, *44*
shirolepa 44
Shiva 9, 18, *18*
shoulders 3, 162
    bones of 82–3, *82*
    massage 168–75, *168–75*, 178, *178*,
        179, *179*
    muscles that move 70–2, *70*
shringatakani marma points *183*, 191,
    191, 195
Shukra Dhatu 18
sinuses 82, 108
    draining 195, *195*
siramatrika marma points 186, *186*
skeletal system 49, 78–85, *78*
skin 59–62, *59*, 149, 163
    problems 62, 109, 129, 132–3
skull 81–2, *81*, 90–1
sleep 220
smiles 208
smoking 219

smooth muscle 66, *67*
smoothing with forearms technique
    174, *174*
snoring 109
sound 24, 39
space/ether 12, 14, 19
sperm 105
spine 43
    postural deformities 84–5, *85*
    spinal column 79–80, *79*
    spinal cord 75
spleen 65
srotas 17
stomach disorders 102, 104, 107, 109
stress 94–5, *95*, 99, 109
    exam 103
    massage for 5, 6, 117
Svadhisthan chakra *31*, *37*, *39*, 197, *197*,
    199
sweat glands 61–2
sweat treatments 44–5
swedana 44–5

talks, giving 240–1
Tamas 156
    tamasic diet 209, *211*
    tamasic mind 26, *27*
    tamasic touch 156
Tantra 18, 19
tapotement 158–9, *158*, 190, *190*
teeth 217–18
telogent hair growth *63*, 64
temperature, high 131
temporomandibular joint (TMJ)
    syndrome 193
tension 3, 4, 5
    see also stress
terminal hair 63
testes 58, 110
therapists 6–7, 143
    appearance 144, *144*
    before and during therapy 165–7
    communication skills 120–2
    ethics 119–20, 145
    posture 145, *145*
    protection 145–7
    see also consultations
thoracic cage 82, *82*
thoracic vertebrae 79, 80
thrombosis 135
thumb pushes 170, *170*, 184, *184*
thumb sweeping technique 168, *168*
thymus gland 58
thyroid glands 57, 59, 104
tinnitus 110

TMJ (temporomandibular joint)
    syndrome 193
tongue 93–4, *94*, 218
touch 91–2, 93, 155, 156
toxins 212, 213, 221, *222*
treatment plans 126
treatment rooms 138–9
    ambience 139–40, *139*
    client care equipment 142–3
    furnishings 142
triclosan 219
trunk, muscles of *72*
turmeric 206

Udana 23
udvartana 45
United States of America
    client confidentiality 236
    insurance 235–6
urinary system 49, 85–7, *85*
usta marma point 192, *192*
uzhichil 45

vajikaran 45
varicose veins 110, 135
VAT (Value Added Tax) 239
Vata *13*, 14, 14–15
    calming oils for 150–1
    colours and 38
    face rejuvenating therapy 203
Vedas 9
veins 51, *51*
vellus hair 62
vertebrae 79–80, *79*
vibrations 161, *161*, 170, *170*, 182, *182*
Vijnanamaya 20, 28
virkurti 12
viruses 152
vishesh 45
Vishudhi chakra *34*, *37*, *39*, 198, *198*, *199*
vitiligo 110
voluntary muscle 66, *67*
Vyana 23

warts 133
water
    in diet 38, 213, 214
    element 11, 15, 29
wellbeing 9
white blood cells 50
wholeness 9, 24
wrinkles 110

Yoga 18–19, 22, 29